THE NEW RULES OF LIFTING FOR WOMEN

THE NEW RULES OF LIFTING FOR WOMEN

Lift Like a Man, Look Like a Goddess

Lou Schuler
with **Cassandra E. Forsythe, M.S.**
Workout programs by **Alwyn Cosgrove**

AVERY
A MEMBER OF PENGUIN GROUP (USA) INC.
NEW YORK

AVERY

Published by the Penguin Group
Penguin Group (USA) Inc., 375 Hudson Street, New York, New York 10014, USA
· Penguin Group (Canada), 90 Eglinton Avenue East, Suite 700, Toronto, Ontario M4P 2Y3, Canada (a division of Pearson Penguin
Canada Inc.) · Penguin Books Ltd, 80 Strand, London WC2R 0RL, England · Penguin Ireland, 25 St Stephen's Green, Dublin 2,
Ireland (a division of Penguin Books Ltd) · Penguin Group (Australia),
250 Camberwell Road, Camberwell, Victoria 3124, Australia (a division of Pearson Australia Group Pty Ltd) · Penguin Books India Pvt
Ltd, 11 Community Centre, Panchsheel Park, New Delhi–110 017, India · Penguin Group (NZ),
67 Apollo Drive, Rosedale, North Shore 0632, New Zealand (a division of Pearson New Zealand Ltd) · Penguin Books (South
Africa) (Pty) Ltd, 24 Sturdee Avenue, Rosebank, Johannesburg 2196, South Africa

Penguin Books Ltd, Registered Offices: 80 Strand, London WC2R 0RL, England

Photography by Michael Tedesco
Illustrations pages 119 and 120 by John Schuler

Most Avery books are available at special quantity discounts for bulk purchase for sales promotions, premiums, fund-raising, and
educational needs. Special books or book excerpts also can be created to fit specific needs.
For details, write Penguin Group (USA) Inc. Special Markets, 375 Hudson Street, New York, NY 10014.

Library of Congress Cataloging-in-Publication Data

Schuler, Lou.
The new rules of lifting for women : lift like a man, look like a goddess / Lou Schuler with Cassandra E. Forsythe ; Workout programs
by Alwyn Cosgrove.
p.   cm.
Includes bibliographical references and index.
ISBN 978-1-58333-294-8
1. Weight lifting.   2. Exercise for women.   I. Forsythe, Cassandra E.   II. Title.
GV546.S35   2007   2007029153
796.41—dc22

Printed in the United States of America
1   3   5   7   9   10   8   6   4   2

BOOK DESIGN BY TANYA MAIBORODA

Acknowledgments

This book exists for one reason. After the original *New Rules of Lifting* was published in January 2006, I received countless e-mails from women asking me why I'd written it for men and ignored their gender entirely. I gave the same reply to many of them: It had never occurred to me to write for any other audience. I'd been fitness editor at *Men's Fitness* and *Men's Health* magazines. My first book was called *The Testosterone Advantage Plan*. I assumed the audience for *New Rules* would be the same one I'd been addressing since 1992.

So for starters, I want to thank the many women who persuaded me to write a book for them.

Second, I want to thank my editor, Megan Newman, a longtime lifter who immediately saw the potential of *The New Rules of Lifting for Women*. Megan went all out to make the book much better than it would've been in the hands of any other editor.

Neither *New Rules* book would have been possible without Alwyn Cosgrove, who designed the workout programs and who has opened my eyes to more great ideas about strength training than anyone else I've worked with.

ACKNOWLEDGMENTS

The "new kid" on this project is Cassandra Forsythe, whom I'd met only once, several years ago, but who enthusiastically jumped aboard when I sent her an e-mail out of the blue to see if she'd be interested in working on this project. Cassandra, a scientist as well as a lifter, inspired and informed this book from beginning to end, and even persuaded her friend Michelle Bower, a strength coach and athlete in Connecticut, to journey to Allentown to act as our model.

Three other contributors made this book possible, as well as a joy to create: my agent, David Black; publicist Gregg Stebben, who more than anyone else is responsible for women's finding out about the original *New Rules of Lifting;* and photographer Michael Tedesco, a longtime colleague whose talent and efficiency made our two-day photo shoot the least stressful of my career.

Thanks also to John Schuler, our illustrator; Mike Mejia, who introduced me to Alwyn; John Berardi, who introduced me to Cassandra; Rebecca Behan at Avery; John Graham and Mike Cerimele at Velocity Sports Performance in Allentown; Mark Verstegen and Amy Wilson at Athletes' Performance; Adam Campbell; and Pete Williams.

I dedicate this book to all the strong women in my life: my mom, Dorothy Schuler, who had biceps before biceps were cool on women; my wife, Kimberly Heinrichs; our younger daughter, Annelise, the family's ballerina; and our older daughter, Meredith—soccer player, skater, climber, and future lifter.   —L.S.

I first want to thank Lou for bringing me in to work on a book that so completely reflects my personal views on diet and exercise. I also want to thank Justin Pribanic, my soul mate, my best friend, and the one man who understands why I work as hard as I do. I'm looking forward to sharing the rest of my life with you.

Thanks to Jeff Volek, my Ph.D. supervisor at the University of Connecticut and the best mentor I could ever hope for.

Finally, I thank my family for loving me and believing in me. This book is for you.
                                                                                 —C.E.F.

Thank you to Derek Campbell, my coach, mentor, and friend. To all the athletes and clients who have trusted me with their bodies, thank you for believing in me. To my friends, colleagues, and teammates over the years, thank you for pushing me to new levels. To the team at Results Fitness, thank you for allowing me to test my theories on you. Thanks to my dad and to my wife, Rachel. And thanks to my mum, who never got the chance to see the lessons she instilled in me take root and bear fruit. This book is for you.
                                                                                 —A.C.

Contents

Introduction:
The Man Show

THE FIRST THING you'll notice about this book is that it's a diet and workout guide for women, written by someone who isn't a woman. In my career as a nonwoman, I've written at least four books for men. (I say "at least" because the concept of authorship can get fuzzy in this genre.) I've been fitness editor at *Men's Fitness* magazine and fitness director at *Men's Health*, and when I wasn't writing for either of those magazines I did some articles for *Men's Journal*. I write a weblog called Male Pattern Fitness, on which I write primarily about health and fitness issues affecting men.

And yet every time I explain the premise of this book to a woman, the reaction is something like this: "Oh, hell yeah!" Or: "About damned time!" Or: "How long do I have to wait?"

Those responses have nothing to do with my charm or good looks—I can produce sworn statements attesting to my deficiencies in both areas—and everything to do with the quality of information about strength training specifically targeted to women.

At a certain point, just about every woman who's ever picked up a dumbbell or walked into a gym reaches the same conclusion: "I'm doing what I'm supposed to be doing, and it isn't working."

The reason:

What you've been told to do *isn't* what you're supposed to do. In the quarter-century since the idea that women could benefit from strength training kicked in, a powerfully counterproductive notion rose in tandem. That's the idea that women should use exercises and techniques different from those used by men.

It's a ridiculous premise, bordering on fraudulence.

And yet every time I walk into a weight room, I see women doing things that nobody would ever recommend to her if she happened to be male. I'll grant you that guys do odd and useless things in the gym as well. (And I'll concede that I take some comfort in that; if they all knew what they were doing, I'd have to find another way to make a living.) Invariably, these women do not appear to be getting the results they should expect from strength training.

Conversely, when I see a woman doing the exercises and using the techniques my coauthors and I recommend, I can see the difference these methods produce in her posture, her confidence in the gym, and the intensity she's able to generate in her workouts. And that's aside from whatever her physique may look like, or how strong she may be. She's probably better than average in both categories, but that doesn't matter. Chances are, she was in a position to learn these exercises and techniques because she was already fit and athletic, with a propensity to gain strength fast.

My point is this: Every woman with a genuine interest in strength training—and here I include anybody who belongs to a gym and uses the weights regularly, or who works out with weights at home—should know how to do the exercises that will help her reach her goals as quickly and efficiently as possible. She should know how to work out in the most productive ways. And she should know these things regardless of her age, physique, or athletic status.

I hope that this book changes your mind about strength exercise in three different ways:

- You'll realize that men and women should be doing workouts that are more similar than different, with women focusing more than they currently do on making their muscles bigger and stronger.
- You'll understand that bigger and stronger muscles will look different on you than they do on me, or anyone else in the nonwoman category.

- You'll see the importance of variety in your workouts, and appreciate the adage that the best workout for you is the one you haven't yet done.

But giving you better workouts, workouts that are constantly challenging you in new and surprising ways, is only half of what my coauthors and I offer you in *The New Rules of Lifting for Women.* We also have a substantial nutrition section, which has three major goals:

- You'll learn that low-calorie diets are a disaster—counterproductive at best, destructive to your long-term health at worst. Some of you will discover that you're eating *too few* calories for your needs. And I think everyone reading *The New Rules of Lifting for Women* will see how dangerous it is to your body, mind, and metabolism to slash the calories in your diet.
- You'll understand why my coauthors and I focus on speeding up your metabolic rate, which is the opposite of the strategy you'll find in typical weight-loss plans.
- You'll see that *when* you eat is more important than *what* you eat. What you eat does matter, of course, which is why we offer plenty of options to make it easy for you to get the right foods at the right times, and in the right amounts. There's no such thing as a perfect diet, but our nutrition guide should help you get as close as possible to an ideal meal plan.

Now, having told you what *New Rules* offers, I should note what you won't find between these covers:

SPECIFIC PROMISES ABOUT HOW MUCH FAT YOU'LL LOSE OR HOW MUCH MUSCLE YOU'LL GAIN

Alwyn Cosgrove, who designed the workout programs, is as highly regarded a fat-loss specialist as anyone in the fitness industry. His clients, male and female, get results that are simply stunning, often with just two workouts a week and dietary modifications. These workouts are based on the ones Alwyn uses in his facility in Santa Clarita, California. Are they the exact same workouts? No. Will you get the same results his clients get? Maybe. You could get better results, or the same, or something less. It's mostly up to you. But I'd be lying if I said that doing workouts without expert supervision is the same as doing them with that kind of guidance.

"BEFORE" AND "AFTER" PICTURES OF PEOPLE WHO'VE DONE THESE PROGRAMS

I've been writing about exercise and nutrition since 1992, and I've never once seen two people get the exact same results from the exact same program. My first book came out in 2002, and since then I've been getting a near-constant stream of feedback from readers of my books who've tried the workouts and used the diet information. The sheer variety of results obtained with the same base of information and advice is staggering. I'll hear from people who tell me they gained double-digit pounds of muscle, or lost scandalous amounts of fat, and they'll be telling me about *the exact same program.* (Not the same diet, obviously.) Sometimes I'll even wonder how they could get better results than I did from a program in one of my own books.

And, in case you're wondering, the opposite sometimes happens as well. I'll hear from a reader who says the programs didn't do anything for him. Actually, I'm lucky if I hear it directly from a reader who has this kind of experience. More often, he shares it with everyone in the form of a negative, and anonymous, review on a website that sells my books. But that's also part of the spectrum of experiences people have with workout programs.

So the first reason for my aversion to before-and-after photos is that they're cherry-picked. They don't really reflect the range of results achieved by readers.

The second reason is that my coauthors and I wrote this book for *you.* It's not about anyone else's results. It's about you achieving your goals. I can't predict how successful you'll be, but I can be damned sure that filling this book with other people's pictures won't help you get there.

MOTIVATIONAL TIPS TO KEEP YOU GOING

As a guy, I'm constitutionally incapable of being perky. I can offer you the best workout plans possible in this format, thanks to Alwyn, and the most up-to-date nutrition advice there is, thanks to coauthor Cassandra Forsythe. I can explain why strength is important, why your metabolism matters, and how to improve both those parameters to help you get the leanest, fittest, healthiest, most age-defying body possible.

I'll even offer online support, on this book's forum at jpfitness.com.

What I can't bring myself to do is find a hundred ways to say "you can do it!" You can do it if you want to do it. I know it. You know it. Do I really need to say it over and over?

Which brings me to the final thing you won't find in these pages:

ANY IMPLICATION THAT YOU, AS A WOMAN, ARE INCAPABLE OF DOING THESE WORKOUTS, OR UNDERSTANDING COMPLEX INFORMATION, AND ACHIEVING THE BEST POSSIBLE RESULTS

This is as good a place as any to hit you with the boring fine print: If you have a medical condition, check with your doctor before jumping into these workouts. We wrote *New Rules* with the idea that you're healthy, and free of orthopedic problems that would affect your ability to do the exercises in this book, and that you don't have allergies to the specific foods we recommend.

If nothing in the boring fine print applies to you, we assume that you can do these workouts, and follow these nutrition plans. You may not be able to do them as well as you'd like, due to coordination or conditioning issues. But those things take care of themselves over time. You get better with practice, and you develop more strength and stamina with time, patience, and effort.

And I say that despite the fact these workouts are not only more challenging than any you'll find that are targeted to women, they're tougher than a lot of the programs designed for men.

I assume you can do them, and benefit from them, because . . . well, because you *can*. Every day, when you get up in the morning, you do things that few people thought a woman could handle a generation or two ago. You probably have a job description that used to apply only to men. You probably have multifaceted responsibilities that no one in my parents' generation thought a woman should ever be expected to do. And yet you're probably doing a workout program that assumes you're weaker-willed and less competent than the average guy in your gym.

I disagree.

If you think I'm right, turn the page, and let's get started.

PART 1

BEHIND THE COVER LINES

Why Should a Woman Lift Like a Man?

IF YOU'VE EVER watched a man working out in a gym, you can be forgiven for not immediately recognizing the bountiful lessons he has to offer. Instead, if you observed anything, it was probably one or more of these:

- poor form
- overly optimistic weight selection, resulting in even poorer form
- odd, guttural noises, usually uttered while lifting too much weight with poor form
- a sudden inability to lift those weights after 8 to 12 repetitions (done with good or bad form), resulting in a pile of iron on the floor and an empty slot on the rack where those weights belong
- a curious attraction to the bench press, which not only results in all of the aforementioned problems, but also is performed with a dedication and zeal that leave no time for exercises designed to work the muscles he can't see in a mirror
- an even more curious lack of awareness that other people can see the muscles that don't show up in his mirror

So what in the world can you learn from the average meathead in your local health club? A lot. I won't pretend that men do anything better than women in the weight room. But I think they understand a few concepts that women tend to ignore. These are by far the most important of all the new rules I'll list in this book.

NEW RULE #1 • The purpose of lifting weights is to build muscle

Weight-training advice for women revolves around what I call the three dirty words: toning, shaping, and sculpting. "Tone," short for "tonus," has a specific meaning in exercise science: it's the firmness of any given muscle when you aren't deliberately flexing it. Tonus improves when you train with weights, but it's not anything you can see.

The way "toning" is used in books and magazines catering to women, and then by women themselves, it means "make your muscles look better without making them bigger." The idea is that there are specific types of workouts—usually involving lots of repetitions with light weights—that will help you achieve this.

But that's not a realistic or healthy way to look at your muscles. If the weights are unchallenging, your muscles won't grow. If your muscles don't grow, they won't look any better than they do now, even if you could somehow strip off whatever fat sits on top of them.

This is such an important point that I'll repeat it:

With or without excess fat, your body simply will not look healthy and fit without well-trained muscle tissue.

"Shaping" offers a different but equally unlikely promise. Muscles can't be "shaped." Their shape is determined by your genetics. You can make them bigger or smaller, and if you're a talented and dedicated bodybuilder you can change their size in proportion to the size of nearby muscles. In other words, you can certainly reshape your body by making some things bigger and other things smaller. But you can't change the shape of individual muscles.

"Sculpting" is the most meaningful of the three words. It implies a combination of muscle growth and fat loss that leaves the lifter's physique looking . . . well, *sculpted.*

But you can't "sculpt" muscles you haven't yet built.

NEW RULE #2 • Muscle is hard to build

When I started lifting weights, back when I was a ridiculously weak and scrawny thirteen-year-old boy who dreaded the humiliation of removing his shirt at the local swimming pool, I dreamed of having muscles roughly the size of the muscles I have now. If you had told me I'd someday be a fairly solid 185-pounder, thanks to the weights, I would've said, "I'm in!"

But if you'd added the caveat that it would take more than three decades to reach that size, I might've had some reservations.

I've never once walked into the gym thinking, "Today I'm going to try to not get too big." For most guys, when we're talking about muscles, there's no such thing as "too big." Those of us who train drug-free celebrate each pound of muscle we add, and every millimeter of upper-arm girth. Some guys even obsess over the circumference of their necks. Why? Because we know that *it's really hard to put on muscle size, it never happens by accident, and every bit of it is a sign of success against all odds.*

And that's with all the hormonal advantages that nature gives to men.

Meanwhile, women, naturally deprived of the amounts of testosterone that would make muscle-building a more straightforward pursuit, worry endlessly about adding so much muscle that they'll turn into the type of shemale you rarely encounter outside *The Howard Stern Show.*

So this brings me to the fourth dirty word: "bulky." As in, "I don't want to get too bulky."

I'll say this as simply as I can:

Unless you're an extreme genetic outlier, you can't get too bulky.

Your body won't allow it. If you put on 10 pounds of muscle in Alwyn's six-month program, you'll be at the top of the class. And if you don't take off at least 10 pounds of fat with the combination of Alwyn's workouts and Cassandra's nutrition plans, I'll be surprised. The most likely outcome, assuming you're willing to work hard, is that you'll come away with a small net loss in body weight, but a dramatic difference in the way your body looks in the mirror and the way your clothes fit. Your tops should be a little tighter, especially in the shoulders, and your trousers a bit roomier, particularly around the waist.

What you don't have to worry about is getting too big. I've been lifting weights longer than many of you have been alive, and I'm still waiting for that moment when I look in the mirror and say, "Damn it, I'm just too big!"

NEW RULE #3 • Results come from hard work

This is a somewhat redundant rule, given that I mentioned hard work in the previous one. But here's something I've observed over my many years of hanging around in gyms: A woman who's willing to work like a galley slave in Spinning class, twist herself into Gordian knots in the yoga studio, and build enough core strength with Pilates to prop up a skyscraper will walk into the weight room, pick up the pastel-colored Barbie weights, and do the exact opposite of what will give her the results she wants.

I'll tell a story that illustrates what I mean:

As I was writing this chapter, I observed a woman at my gym doing two exercises in combination. The first was triceps kickbacks, a simple and useless exercise in which you lean over a bench, hold your upper arm parallel to the floor, and straighten your elbow while holding a very light weight. The second was one-arm rows, in which you lean over a bench with your upper arm perpendicular to the floor, and row the weight up to the side of your abdomen.

A rowing exercise involves far more muscles, including the lats and trapezius, the big, strong muscles of the upper back. Plus, since it's a multijoint exercise, the muscles that bend the elbow, such as the biceps, are also involved. And in addition to all that, the leverage on a one-arm row is perfect for lifting relatively heavy weights—you have one foot on the floor, and the opposite knee and hand braced on the bench. There's no stress on your lower back, and it's not unusual to see serious bodybuilders doing this exercise with a dumbbell weighing 100 pounds or more.

The kickback, meanwhile, is an awkward exercise, with relatively poor leverage. The only movement is at the elbow joint, which is not designed to move heavy weights at that angle. Even a beginner would probably be able to use three or four times as much weight on a row versus a kickback.

This woman was using 6-pound dumbbells for the kickbacks . . . and 7-pound weights for the rows.

I asked a trainer at the gym if he'd seen what I'd just seen. He shook his head sadly, and said that the toughest part of his job was getting women to use weights heavy enough to make their time in the gym worthwhile.

So even if a woman understands the first two rules in this chapter—that the object of lifting is to build muscle, and that muscle is hard to build—the idea that she truly needs to challenge herself in the weight room may not get through.

NEW RULE #4 • Hard work includes lifting heavier weights

It's not enough to progress from lifting the Barbie 'bells fifteen times to lifting them twenty times. It may be an accomplishment—that is, the result of purposeful and exhausting work—but it's not going to make muscles bigger. Muscles grow for a variety of reasons, but the main one is strength. If you force them to get stronger, they will get bigger. If you start lifting 100 pounds five times, but train your body to lift 150 pounds five times, you're going to end up with bigger muscles. But if you start off lifting 50 pounds ten times, and progress to lifting the same 50 pounds fifteen times, all you've done is increase the endurance of the muscles, which by itself will not make them bigger.

NEW RULE #5 • From time to time, you have to break some of the old rules

You'll rarely see a woman lifting weights with bad form in a gym. And you'll almost always see at least one man slinging iron around with technique so miserably wrong you want to dial 9 and 1 on your cell phone just to save time when the inevitable spine-buckling accident occurs.

In between the extremes, you'll see lots of guys pushing themselves out to the edge of acceptable form to get an extra repetition in their final set of an exercise, or to hit a new personal record on a lift. If nothing else, you'll probably see guys lift at a variety of speeds, perhaps shifting into a faster gear near the end of a set to help them complete more repetitions. The more experienced a male lifter is, the more he learns to trust his own body and his own instincts. (Alas, inexperienced lifters often feel the same way, even if their instincts haven't yet earned that trust.)

But you'll rarely see a woman deviate from the textbook description of the exercise. And when it comes to the tempo of her lifts, she performs them like clockwork, even if it means she has to use unchallenging weights to make such precision possible.

I'd never advocate lifting with bad form. But there's more to strength training than coloring inside the lines.

Part of the problem is fear. When women are introduced to the weight room, they're taught that there's only one way to perform each exercise, and that small adjustments to accommodate individual biomechanics will put her in the ER. If anybody tries to instill such fear in a man, the sound magically stops before it reaches his eardrums.

To make things worse, women are sometimes presented with cautions that have little basis in the real world, creating fear of injury when the actual risk is nonexistent.

For example, in the book *Body for Life for Women,* the author offers this instruction for a simple shoulder press: "Press the weights up until your arms are almost straight (with your elbows just short of locked)." Since the author is Pamela Peeke, M.D., and not some garden-variety personal trainer or celebrity who decided to expand her investment portfolio by writing a workout book, you'd assume the anti-elbow-straightening precaution has a basis in science. That is, straightening your arms at the elbow joints must be bad for you.

It's not.

In all my years of writing about strength training, and in all my months of studying for my credentials as a trainer, I've never come across any suggestion of injury risk from this simple movement. More to the point, elbows are *supposed* to lock. It's called "straightening your arms." The triceps muscles are designed to straighten your elbows until they reach that locked position. If you don't lock, you don't work your triceps through their full range of motion, which means you don't get the full benefits of the elbow-straightening exercise you're performing.

My issue here isn't with the idea that people should exercise with caution, and I'm not arguing for more reckless abandon in the weight room. What I am saying is that your body has natural movement patterns, which support a range of variations.

Maybe all strength-training precautions can be reduced to these two sentences:

If it's what your body was designed to do, it's probably not bad form. And if the exercise requires you to do something unnatural, you should think twice before doing it.

How to Feel Like a Natural Woman

I realize that the word "natural" isn't always helpful in early twenty-first-century America, where humans spend much of the day sitting at desks or driving cars, two actions that no one would argue our bodies evolved to perform. To me, a "natural" position or movement is one you would assume or perform in an athletic activity.

Picture yourself playing volleyball, getting ready to return the other team's serve. Your feet are parallel to each other, perhaps shoulder-width apart, with toes pointed forward. Your knees are bent slightly. (You'd never play any sport with stiff knees; you'd be virtually immobile.) Your lower back is arched slightly. Your shoulders are square, and your midsection's tight. That's what a human body looks like when it's ready for physical action, whether that action is a game, a hunt, or a wrestling match.

Now picture a typical woman standing at the cable station in a typical gym, getting ready to perform triceps extensions. (In case you're new to lifting, the extension is an elbow-straightening exercise, usually done with a straight bar attached to the cable.) Her feet are together, her knees are locked, her lower back is flat, and her shoulders are hunched up toward her ears. In other words, she's in the opposite of an athletic position, despite the fact she's about to do an exercise that, in theory, will make her body more athletic.

NEW RULE #6 • No workout will make you taller

Workout advice for women is riddled with allusions to making muscles "longer." I started noticing it a few years ago at the front end of the Pilates craze. In fact, I was on a panel at a conference with an editor from a women's magazine who, in discussing fitness trends, said that women didn't want to build "bulky" muscles; instead, they wanted "long, lean muscles, like a dancer's," and they could get these muscles from Pilates. I started laughing (not my most gracious moment, I admit), and wondered if I should start telling my readers at *Men's Health* that our workouts could make them taller. The poor woman looked stunned; I don't think it had occurred to her that her pro-Pilates sentiments were nothing more than propaganda.

The reality is this: muscles, as aforementioned, have a genetically predetermined shape. If you train and feed a muscle so that it grows, you can't choose whether the muscle becomes "bulky" or "long and lean, like a dancer's," any more than you can choose your own height. I won't claim men are inherently reality-based—I've gotten e-mails from more than one guy asking how he can get "ripped abs, like Brad Pitt" (my answer: "For starters, you'll need his parents")—but I've never had anyone ask me how he can make his muscles "longer." It just doesn't occur to guys to think of their bodies as being that malleable.

That said, I think both genders fall for the entirely fallacious notion that by doing a particular person's workout, they can have a physique like that person. Anyone in the business of publishing bodybuilding magazines will tell you that the surest way to sell more copies than usual is to slap a black-and-white picture of Arnold Schwarzenegger on the cover, and promise Schwarzeneggerian results with the workout routine inside. For some reason, it never occurs to anyone that Arnold was the only guy in the history of bodybuilding who ever looked like Arnold. Logically, that suggests a one-of-a-kind quirk in Schwarzenegger's genetic code, something that allowed him to achieve unique physical proportions that were simply unattainable by anyone else.

Same goes for whichever model or actress is on the cover of *Shape* or *Fitness* or *Self* this month. You can use their "Exclusive Stay-Slim Workout Secrets!" from now till doomsday, but there's not a chance in a million you'll emerge with a belly, shank, or rump like that celebrity unless your genetics allow it.

Another idea I'd like to dispel, while I'm at it:

Let's say you accept the impossibility of developing a celebrity's proportions without being a clone of that celebrity. Chances are, you still believe that you can achieve a "type" of physique if you train like people who have that type. Magazines feed this notion, rarely stated in so many words, by showing tall, lean models doing workouts that promise readers a long, lean physique.

Of course, this makes perfect sense from the magazines' point of view. They aren't going to sell many copies if they show short, chunky women in their workout features. But you have to understand that the models doing the workouts are just that. They were cast by the photo editors specifically because they already have what the feature promises. If the exercises in the feature are unique, you can bet the model is doing them for the first time. She had that body when she walked in the door of the photo studio, and she'll still have it when she walks out. That's why she's a model.

An obvious point? Okay. But raise your hand if you believe that running will make you look like a runner. If your hand isn't in the air, you're probably not being honest with yourself. Don't you believe that running makes you lose weight, and that successful runners are skinny because they run? Isn't that why you, or people you know, turn to endurance exercise as the first step in a weight-loss program?

I'm not going to tackle the myths and realities of long-distance locomotion until Chapter 3, and I won't for a second argue that women are more susceptible to the seductive strains of "Build a Dancer's Body!" than men are to the testosterone-soaked dream of "Build Arms Like Arnold's!"

But if we don't start this relationship with a firm grasp of the reality of our undertaking, it's just not going to work. And if it doesn't work, you'll go right back to toning, shaping, and sculpting, not to mention living in fear of being bulky. Even worse, if things really go bad, I may have to go back to writing articles about Brad Pitt's abs. Nobody wants that.

The Truth About
Your Muscles

ANYBODY WITH EYES and ears can recite the differences between men and women. Women are smaller, on average, and have higher-pitched voices. And some key differences exist beyond what's immediately visible. Adult women will tend to have a higher proportion of fat and a lower proportion of muscle mass, compared with men. They also have slower metabolic rates, smaller hearts and lungs relative to body size, shorter legs, and narrower shoulders. With that out of the way, it's time to rule.

NEW RULE #7 • Muscles in men and women are essentially identical

A muscle fiber in a woman isn't structurally different from a muscle fiber in a man. There are some chemical differences, due to the need to interact with different hormones at the cell-membrane level, but those aspects don't change a fiber's functional abilities. We may be separate genders, but we aren't separate species.

NEW RULE #8 • Muscle strength is a matter of life and death

Health improves with increased strength and muscle mass, and that's just as true for women as it is for men.

Consider this: In a study of elderly women who were disabled to varying degrees, researchers for the U.S. National Institute on Aging found that those with the least strength were twice as likely to die from heart disease as the strongest. The researchers on that study, published in 2003, used hand-grip strength as a measure of total strength.

A University of Pittsburgh study published in 2006 looked at an additional measure of strength—testing the quadriceps (the muscles on the front of your thighs)—and found a similar effect. The weakest women had 1.65 times the risk of death from any cause, compared to the strongest.

Of course, you aren't elderly or disabled. I use those examples to prove a point: Strength has very real implications for your quality of life—your *entire* life. And although strength isn't perfectly correlated with muscle size (obese people tend to have a lot of muscle mass, which they need to haul the extra fat they're carrying from one room to the next), it's a pretty good way to determine how well your muscles are working.

I have two goals in this chapter. The first is to look at what we know about helping women increase their strength and muscle size, and the second is to examine the small but real differences in men and women that will affect the outcome of your exercise programs.

WHAT'S GOOD FOR THE GANDER . . .

As far back as 1986, a study in the journal *Sports Medicine* asked whether women should do the same workout routines as men, and came to this conclusion: "Very little difference is seen in the response to different modes of progressive-resistance strength training." In 1990, in the same journal, two researchers noted this: "Unit for unit, female muscle tissue is similar in force output to male muscle tissue. . . . There is no evidence that women should train differently [from how men do]."

Translating that into English, what the researchers are saying is that the muscles of a woman are capable of performing similarly to those of a man. Because women's muscles are smaller, a typical woman's absolute strength will be less than that of a typical man. But there's nothing a man's muscles can do that a woman's can't.

The technical term for muscles' ability to generate strength and power is "muscle quality." But a better term for this conversation might be "muscle equality." As in, when you control for the size of the muscles of the people you're testing, there's no important difference in the genders. Studies generally show that men are a bit stronger, muscular pound for muscular pound, but the difference falls into the range of 5 to 10 percent.

GETTING HYOOOGE!

Here's something else I'll bet you didn't know: Women and men increase muscle and strength at roughly the same rate in the same training programs. That doesn't mean a woman will gain as much muscle as a man; she'll just make the same percentage increases as her male counterpart.

Let's say you have two young adults who're relative novices in the weight room. He weighs 200 pounds, with 20 percent of that in the form of fat. That means he has 160 pounds of lean mass. The woman weighs 120 pounds, with 30 percent body fat. (Yeah, they've both kind of let themselves go.) So she has 90 pounds of lean mass.

They both do the same six-month workout program. Since the program is designed by Alwyn, they both increase their lean mass—mostly in the form of muscle—by 10 percent. His 10 percent weighs 16 pounds, a spectacular success. His shoulders are wider, his chest muscles do a little dance when he moves his arms, and his upper arms threaten to demolish the sleeves of his golf shirts. He vows to name his firstborn son Alwyn, even though he's not quite sure how to pronounce it. (For the record, it's "ALL-in.")

She, meanwhile, gains 9 pounds of lean mass. Her reaction is . . . well, to tell you the truth, she's excited, too. That's because those 9 pounds of muscle don't look anything like the 16 pounds of muscle added by her male counterpart. Her shoulders are certainly wider, which she's happy about, knowing the straps of her sundresses will finally stay on her shoulders this summer, instead of sliding off. Her arms are a tiny bit thicker, with visible ripples in her triceps and an emerging biceps bump right above her elbow. But her thighs have only increased a third of an inch in circumference, and in exchange for that small gain in size she has quadriceps that look like they were carved out of stone, rather than fudge ripple ice cream. Her waist is actually a half inch smaller.

And whereas the bulked-up man now weighs 212 pounds (having lost 4 pounds of fat while gaining four times that in muscle), Our Lady of the Weight Room still weighs 120 pounds. It's not the same 120 pounds, of course; she's now at 17.5 percent body fat, with new curves and contours everywhere she looks.

You may think I'm making up those numbers and, in fact, I am . . . kind of. The upper limit of muscle gain for women is about two and a half pounds per month, so I picked a number that was between half and two-thirds of that. And the circumference measurements came directly from a variety of studies conducted between the mid-1970s and the mid-1990s.

Some of those studies show a concurrent increase in muscle size and reduction in body fat. I can't possibly guarantee that it'll happen for you specifically—as the ads say, "individual results may vary"—but it has been shown to happen. Sometimes it happens in the exact same places. You can't call it spot reduction, where you exercise a specific region of your body with the goal of shrinking the fat in that area. (This doesn't work, as you probably know.) But, since women will tend to lose fat first in their arms and bellies during a serious exercise program, they end up exhibiting a phenomenon you could call "spot substitution"—gaining muscle in their upper arms, for example, while also losing fat there. You can't predict or train for a one-to-one exchange of muscle for fat, but in some studies it appears to have worked out that way.

One of the researchers even took pictures to illustrate the point. William Kraemer, Ph.D., probably the most influential strength-training researcher of my lifetime, used magnetic resonance imaging (MRI) to show women's arms and legs before and after training programs. The MRIs allow you to see the increase in muscle and decline in fat after twelve weeks, with only minor changes in the girth of those limbs.

Different studies have shown different results, as you can imagine. Sometimes fat decreases with no increase in muscle, which means the circumferences of the arms or legs or waist or whatever's measured will decline. Sometimes the opposite happens, and muscle increases without a loss of fat. (This is most likely to happen in the lower body, where initial fat loss is usually slow when compared to the upper body; that's why you need the combination of Cassandra's diet plans and Alwyn's workouts to tip the balance.) But in no studies I've seen have women's measurements increased more than a fraction of an inch due to muscle gain, and in many studies everything that was measured decreased. The one exception is shoulder width. Getting stronger and adding upper-body muscle tissue will almost certainly widen your shoulders. But unless you're a runway model, it's hard to see any aesthetic or functional downside to having wider, more athletic-looking shoulders. Your neck will look longer and your waist and hips will look smaller. If anyone considers those negative consequences, it's news to me.

BIG GIRLS, SMALL FIBERS

My overwhelming memory of life before puberty is a general one of being so skinny that the prepubescent girls in my class had bigger arms, legs, and shoulders. I assume that changed when our hormones kicked in, but it's hard to say. Frankly, I can't recall ever checking out the girls' arm girth past the age of twelve. There were just too many visual distractions by then.

I bring up my prepuberty physique, and yours, for a reason:

Muscle fibers fall into two broad categories—type I, the ones responsible for endurance-type movement, and type II, the ones associated with strength and power. The fibers of your girl muscles and my boy muscles were about the same size before my voice changed and yours didn't. Your type I fibers, as well as mine, were actually larger than your type IIs, even though type II fibers have much more potential for growth.

Then, while you were learning to shave your legs, something interesting began to happen in mine. All my muscle fibers began to grow, but my type II fibers began to grow *a lot*. If I were an average young man, and you were an average young woman, type I fibers would make up about 36 percent of the total muscle mass in my legs. But they'd take up 44 percent of the space occupied by muscle in yours. (I'm talking about the size of fibers here, not the number of them or their distribution. Men and women have roughly equal numbers of muscle fibers and percentages of each type of fiber.)

That means almost two-thirds of my muscle mass consists of type II fibers, the ones that allow me to sprint, jump, lift heavy weights, or throw things really hard. You, on the other hand, have just more than half of your muscle tissue devoted to those feats of strength and power.

Moreover, your type I fibers tend to be bigger than your type IIs; it's the opposite in men.

I know this seems really technical and geeky, but trust me, I'm building up to an important point here: Women typically start out in a training program with type I fibers—the ones designed for endurance—that are not just bigger than your type II fibers, but that also take up almost half the space in your muscles.

Since this information is well-known, it's often misinterpreted by trainers to mean that women should emphasize endurance over strength when they work out. You'll often see trainers have their female clients do sets of 15 or more repetitions, because, the reasoning goes, women are inherently better at exercises that require endurance, so programs should emphasize that quality.

The problem with that is something Alwyn has said on many occasions: "If you do what you've always done, you get what you've always gotten."

The ideal strategy should be the reverse of the conventional "do lots of reps because women are good at that." Because women start out with type II fibers that are relatively smaller, they may actually have greater potential to make those fibers bigger, compared to men. I say "may" because it's hardly a settled issue. Different studies look at different muscles in different ways and report different results. But nobody believes that women have *less* potential to develop their type II fibers, which brings me to this corollary of New Rules 1 through 4:

The goal in the weight room is to develop type II muscle fibers, which have the greatest potential for growth.

THE BETTER HALF

Women have some advantages over men in the weight room—or in any type of training, for that matter. For one thing, your muscles recover faster. They regenerate ATP, the chemical that provides the energy for muscle actions, faster than male muscles.

You also experience less muscle soreness in the day or two after workouts. So if you and I do the same workout, and neither of us is accustomed to the exercises or the level of intensity, you'll feel the post-exercise soreness faster than I will, but I'll feel the pain longer, and it'll seem more dramatic to me than it does to you. (It doesn't exactly make up for childbirth, but it's still a win for your team.)

That's why Alwyn's workouts in *The New Rules of Lifting for Women* are actually a bit more challenging than the ones he designed for men in our previous collaboration. You can take it.

One last man-woman thing:

Women will probably experience a bit more inflammation after a tough workout than will men. It sounds bad, but it isn't. An inflammatory response means you got your muscles' attention by inducing some minor damage, which your body has to repair. That cycle of damage and repair is the key to building bigger, stronger muscles, and may also be a reason why strength training speeds up your metabolism. Everything in your body has to work harder to shore up those (slightly) damaged muscles. The idea is to make sure your body is ready for the workout the next time you do it. If your internal repair team is doing its job, that same workout won't create the same inflammatory response the second time around. Which brings me to this:

NEW RULE #9 • A muscle's "pump" is not the same as muscle growth

Inflammation can make muscles feel bigger, even though the only thing that's grown is the amount of fluid your muscles are holding, and that's temporary. But I should warn you that some women have been known to interpret that transitory swelling as proof that they're "bulking up," which absolutely is not what's going on. It takes weeks for actual, measurable muscle growth to occur, no matter how tight your arms or legs feel the day after one of Alwyn's workouts.

Men and women tend to react differently to post-workout inflammation. Both of us will misinterpret the fluid buildup as proof that our muscles are getting bigger, but while you will worry that you're turning into Hulkette, I'll strut around like I've suddenly morphed into the "after" picture in a supplement ad. You might overreact by turning down the intensity of future workouts, which will undermine your goals, but my reaction could be even worse. I'll try to produce that inflammation after every workout as proof that my muscles are still growing, and I'll end up overtraining. At best, the result will be that I won't have anything to show for all my sweat and tears, since I'm not allowing my body to recover from one workout to the next. At worst, I'll get hurt, burn out, or become one of those guys who post too much on Internet bodybuilding forums.

Consider this fair warning: You may feel sore after some of Alwyn's workouts, particularly when you jump into a new phase of the program, with exercises and protocols you haven't tried before. You may even notice some swelling and tightness in your muscles. Just remember that these are signs that the program is working, not that it's working too well.

Step Away from the Treadmill

THIS IS THE PART of the book where you start to wonder if maybe I'm the victim of too many protein shakes. I'm going to argue that steady-pace endurance exercise—what most of us refer to as "cardio" or "aerobics"—is overrated as a tool for fat loss. But before I do, let me point out that I'm not disputing any of the facts that are indisputable. Does endurance exercise burn calories? Sure. Does it contribute to a longer, healthier life? Absolutely.

I'm not out to demonize anyone's favorite type of exercise. I just want to show you a better way to lose body fat, and I want to alleviate any fear you might have that *not* doing endurance exercise will somehow make you less healthy. (See "The Heart of the Matter" on page 27 for a detailed look at exercise and heart health.) Alwyn's workouts call for plenty of exercise, including exercise at high levels of intensity, which will give you all the benefits you want from endurance exercise without actually requiring much of it. The "higher levels of intensity" is crucial, as I'll explain in detail throughout this chapter.

NEW RULE #10 • Endurance exercise is an option, not a necessity, for fat loss

Okay, I said it: You don't need to do any endurance work, if you don't want. Alwyn's female clients typically lose fat rapidly, with or without it. That's because the two most powerful drivers of fat loss are diet and anaerobic exercise. I'll get into diet in the next section, and stick with exercise in this chapter, although I'll warn you that there's going to be some crossover. We aren't proposing that you do Alwyn's workouts without changing your diet, or that you follow Cassandra's nutrition plan without also building some sweat equity in the weight room. Frankly, we don't know how well either component works without the other.

NEW RULE #11 • "Aerobics" doesn't mean what you think it means

Dr. Kenneth Cooper, a former college track star, coined the word "aerobics" to promote endurance exercise. Here's what he wrote in *Aerobics,* his 1968 best seller: "I'll state my position early. The best exercises are running, swimming, cycling, walking, stationary running, handball, basketball, and squash, and in just about that order. Isometrics, weight lifting, and calisthenics, though good as far as they go, don't even make the list, despite the fact that most exercise books are *based* on one of these three."

Cooper believed that steady-pace exercise was the key to everything. It was a counterintuitive idea, but unlike so many other leap-of-faith notions that arose in the 1960s ("Tune in, turn on, drop out"), it gained a permanent foothold in science and practice. I call it "counterintuitive" because the human species didn't really evolve to excel at long-distance runs. We're made to *walk* long distances—that's how our ancient ancestors put food on the table, before they figured out retailing—and to run really fast when we must. We're good at start-stop activities involving lots of different speeds and changes of direction, which is why human children instinctively play games like "tag," why human adults invent games like basketball and soccer, and why fighting sports like boxing and tae kwon do have rounds of several minutes, rather than continuous action until one fighter wins.

What most of us aren't good at, by nature, is jogging or swimming at a steady pace for longer than a few minutes.

And yet that's what Cooper and many who followed his example have spent four decades telling us we should do.

To be fair, it's hard to make the argument that we're designed to do sets of bench presses or deadlifts, either. So maybe it's facetious to take any aspects of modern life, including our exercise routines, and put them into a prehistoric context. I'm just trying to make the point that the ability to do anaerobic exercises—lifting heavy things, running fast, jumping, climbing, fighting—was vital to the survival of our species. Being able to jog for an hour at a specified percentage of your maximum heart rate wasn't.

The word "aerobic" refers to the aerobic energy system, one of three ways your body can fuel movement. You use your aerobic system constantly, whether you think about it or not. As long as you're breathing easily, whether you're working, sleeping, doing chores, or exercising, you're using it. That is, you're using oxygen to burn a combination of fat and glycogen (the form of carbohydrate your body uses for energy) to keep your body functioning.

Generally, the healthier you are, the higher the percentage of fat you'll burn at rest. If you're obese and/or diabetic, you'll burn more glycogen and less fat. A perfectly healthy woman would burn just under 60 percent fat and just over 40 percent glycogen most of the time. During exercise, as your heart rate quickens and you start breathing harder, the ratio will shift. All-out exercise is anaerobic—your body can't use oxygen to burn fuel, so it uses chemicals inside your body to generate the energy it needs. When your body needs to fuel movement without oxygen, it uses glycogen, rather than fat, to keep you moving. It has two systems for this: one for very short sprints, up to perhaps ten seconds, and the other for longer dashes that last about a minute.

Given what I just wrote, you'd think that exercising with the aerobic energy system must be superior to using either of your two anaerobic systems, since you burn more fat with aerobics. That's where we got the now-very-much-discredited idea that there's a "fat-burning zone" in which we should all exercise.

The amount of fat you burn during exercise matters less than the amount you burn when you aren't exercising. And that's where you start to see some of the hidden benefits of strength training.

KILLER CALORIES

If you compare the number of calories burned during endurance exercise with the number burned during strength training, endurance wins pretty easily. Let's say you weigh 140 pounds. If you ran five miles in an hour—a twelve-minute-mile pace—

you'd burn an estimated 512 calories. (That's including the 100 or so calories you'd burn in that hour if you didn't go running, but that's the same no matter what type of exercise we're looking at.) An hour of serious strength training would burn an estimated 384 calories, or 25 percent fewer. If you're a talented runner clocking eight-minute miles, you'd burn 800 calories, or more than twice as many as you'd burn in the weight room for that same hour.

At first glance, it's easy to see why strength training doesn't slay calories the way endurance exercise does. You spend more time resting in between sets than you do actually lifting, and you certainly aren't burning fat while you're pushing and pulling weights. If you're challenging yourself at all, you're shifting from your fat-using aerobic energy system to your anaerobic systems, which by design run on glycogen.

However, there is more going on.

First is the afterburn—the calories your body continues to burn after the workout is over. Intensity is the most important factor determining post-workout metabolism, so the harder you work in the weight room, the more calories your body will burn afterward. Let's say that afterburn accounts for an additional 50 calories.

Calories aren't the only consideration. Serious strength training also signals your body to burn a higher percentage of fat calories for many hours after you leave the gym. An intriguing University of Colorado study, published in the *Journal of Applied Physiology* in 2003, measured post-workout fat oxidation. ("Fat oxidation" is what happens when your body uses oxygen to turn fat into energy, as it does when you're using your aerobic energy system.) The researchers had a group of men and women do a weight workout one day and an aerobic workout another, with each workout burning about 400 calories.

Fifteen hours after the weight workout, the men and women were burning 22 percent more fat than they did fifteen hours after their aerobic workout. The researchers concluded that the exercisers would've needed to burn twice as many calories during their aerobic workout—800, instead of 400—to reach the level of post-workout fat oxidation achieved by the lifters.

"BURN MORE CALORIES WHILE YOU SLEEP!"

I haven't yet mentioned resting metabolic rate (RMR), which is the speed at which your body burns calories regardless of whatever you happen to be doing at the moment. With men, it's pretty clear that weight lifting increases RMR. The workouts themselves speed up metabolism, in part because the body needs to work harder to repair and rebuild muscles, connective tissues, and bones. And then there's a cumulative effect that comes from adding new muscle tissue. It isn't anything close to the "50 calories per pound of muscle" that some people claim (and I say that knowing full well I've used that figure in articles going back a few years). But muscle is metabolically active tissue, and having more of it certainly forces your body to burn more calories throughout the day and night. The real key, though, is the workouts. The harder they are, the more calories you burn in the next day or two as your body recovers.

Unfortunately, it's difficult to make any of these claims with women. Some studies have shown a metabolic boost from strength training, and some haven't. Here are two examples:

A study conducted at Colorado State University, published in 2000, showed that resting metabolic rates of young women were still elevated by 4.2 percent sixteen hours after lifting weights. It was a small study, with just seven women between twenty-two and thirty-five years old.

But a University of Maryland study, published the next year, showed that women had no chronic increase in their metabolic rates after a twenty-four-week strength-training program. That study used two groups of women—nine who were in their twenties, and ten who were over sixty-five. There is a slight twist to this conclusion: The researchers found no *statistically significant* increase, but the women were in fact burning about 50 extra calories a day after six months of training. That was an increase of close to 4 percent. The men in the same study increased their metabolic rates by about 9 percent, so the women's gains, even if they had been large enough to pass statistical muster, were still a fraction of the men's.

I do think it's worth noting, though, that the significant metabolic increase in one study and the insignificant increase in the other aren't so far apart. True, the two studies looked at separate issues—elevated metabolism the day after a workout versus resting metabolic rate removed from the context of a recent workout—but they showed something similar. Women do seem to get a slight increase in metabolism from lifting. It's still in the neighborhood of just 50 calories a day, which isn't even a fifth of a Snickers bar. But it shows that the weights are doing something that probably won't happen with endurance exercise.

So if you add it all up, weight workouts give you two, and possibly three, important advantages over endurance exercise:

1. The afterburn, which might be an extra 50 calories.
2. A higher percentage of fat calories used for energy after the workout.

3. A possible increase in resting metabolic rate, in the neighborhood of 50 calories a day.

Having said all that, I'll acknowledge that you could equal these benefits of resistance training simply by doing more endurance exercise, or doing it at a higher intensity. You'd burn more calories, you'd get a greater afterburn than you would by exercising at an easier pace, and you'd train your body, over time, to use a higher percentage of fat calories during your runs or swims or rides, and to tap into those fat stores earlier in the workout.

Can strength training compete with that? Let me explain why I think the answer is yes.

THE POWER OF PERTURBATION

Let's slow down for a moment, and ask ourselves why strength training has a bigger effect on metabolism and post-exercise fat-burning than endurance exercise. I think there are two key reasons.

First, there's the inefficiency factor. When you hear your boss use a word like "inefficiency," you know someone in the office will soon be using monster.com as her home page, and you hope it's not you. But when we talk about inefficient exercise, we're talking about routines that require more effort. Your body isn't used to the exercises yet, or hasn't fully adapted to the exercise parameters, and thus has to work harder to get through the routine. Harder work means better results—you'll burn more calories during the workout, and you'll burn more afterward, when your body is recovering. In other words, inefficiency is the ideal.

The problem with a repetitive routine, like running or cycling, is that your body makes adaptations and gets progressively more efficient. Those adaptations allow you to go farther and faster in your runs or rides, which is good if your goal is to be an endurance athlete who goes farther and faster. If your goal is to be leaner, then greater endurance isn't really to your benefit; the increased efficiency means you use fewer calories per unit of exercise.

Here's a study that illustrates the problem:

Back in 1990, researchers at the U.S. Department of Agriculture published a study that compared the effects of diet and exercise versus exercise alone for overweight women. The diet was extreme, cutting the women's daily calorie intake by 50 percent. Both groups of women did six days a week of steady-pace endurance exercise, thirty-five to forty minutes a day. The diet-plus-exercise group lost a boatload of weight, as you can imagine—29 pounds in twelve weeks, on average. Unfortunately, a third of it was muscle, which meant their resting metabolic rates slowed down by an average of 9 percent. The exercise group also lost weight, about 13 pounds per person, but only 14 percent of it was lean tissue, and their metabolic rates stayed the same. But the really, really startling finding is that the first group became so efficient at endurance exercise that they burned 16 percent fewer calories when doing it at low intensities. The exercise group also got more efficient, but only burned 8 percent fewer calories. (I should note that the effect disappeared at higher intensities of exercise, which gets back to what I said earlier about the importance of working harder versus longer.)

One more negative effect of chronic endurance exercise:

Your body will adapt to the increased efficiency by selectively shrinking your type I muscle fibers. Yes, literally, those fibers get smaller as they get better at running or riding. The effect may not be dramatic, but it illustrates how endurance exercise makes your body more efficient, which is to say better at going longer distances with less fuel. If you're trying to get your body to burn *more* fuel, you can see the problem here.

The same problem arises with strength training, if you forget the "strength" and focus on the "training." Doing high-repetition work with light weights simply makes your muscles more efficient at lifting light weights, which is a surefire way to shrink your muscles and reduce their ability to burn calories.

Heavier lifts, as you can imagine, are inherently less efficient than lighter lifts. They require a bit more energy to perform, but consume a lot more energy as your body recovers from them.

Imagine a lower-body workout that includes leg presses versus one in which you do squats with a barbell on your shoulders. For the leg press, you're merely straightening your legs by pushing on a platform that, by virtue of its 45-degree angle, is designed to be easy to push. Contrast that with barbell squats, in which most of your body's muscle fibers are involved in either lifting the weight or keeping your body upright while you lift it. The squatting movement is natural—we do it every time we jump or get up from a chair—but the heavy weight and the difficulty of keeping it balanced on your shoulders make it extraordinarily inefficient.

That inefficiency flips all the switches on what's called your sympathetic nervous system. Again, forget that the word "sympathetic" has warm and fuzzy connotations in most of its uses. When we're talking about our nervous system, "sympathetic" involves the heavy-duty stuff, the stress hormones that trigger our fight-or-flight responses. It's your body's internal equivalent of a smoke detector.

Activating the sympathetic nervous system means your adrenal glands are kicking out adrenaline and other stress hormones, your heart rate and blood pressure increase, and your bronchial passages widen. Your body's core temperature increases, your sweat glands open, your pupils dilate, and you might even get goose bumps.

We're conditioned to think that all these things are bad, but in the context of a workout, they're actually good, since without this festival of stress, you wouldn't be able to work as hard in the weight room. And your body wouldn't burn as many calories, or use as much fat for energy, while you're recovering.

In other words, the real key to successful strength training is *metabolic perturbation*. You're shaking things up in your muscle cells, your nervous system, and your hormones. The calories you burn while throwing so much of your body into the spin cycle can be modest or substantial, but they're only part of the effect. What your body does afterward, when it's trying to recover, has at least as big an impact on your physique as the calories used while you're actually lifting.

Could you shake things up with endurance exercise? Sure, if you do intervals, which are a mix of all-out and easy efforts, rather than running or riding at a steady pace. But at that point, you're shifting away from your exclusive use of your aerobic energy system and using one or both of your anaerobic systems. In other words, you've stopped doing "aerobics" and started doing something that resembles strength training, at least in terms of energy. You're selectively using glycogen-fueled movement with the goal of forcing your body to use more fat while it recovers.

And that's exactly what Alwyn wants you to do.

Retrofitting Your Genes

This is as good a place as any to emphasize something that books like this usually ignore: the way your genes influence your results. Those who study weight loss acknowledge that no two people will process calories the exact same way, unless those people are identical twins.

If you set out to compose a list of every exercise- and diet-related variable that's genetically dependent, you'd start with these:

- strength
- aerobic capacity

- body-fat percentage
- body-fat distribution
- spontaneous physical activity (how much you move on any given day)
- how many calories you burn during digestion (a phenomenon I'll address in the next chapter)
- resting metabolic rate

Different studies attach different numbers to all those variables, but most seem to settle into the range of 30 to 40 percent. So when you lift, for example, your genes probably determine about 30 to 40 percent of the results you get. When you diet, your genes weigh in on how your body reacts—how much fat you lose, where the fat comes off, the degree to which your metabolism slows down.

But here's a cool fact to know: Exercise intensity trumps genetics. The harder you work, the less influence your genes have on the results of that work. The tipping point seems to be when you're working at a pace that requires six times the energy you'd use at rest, which researchers abbreviate as "6 METs." (For a list of exercises and activities and their MET values, see the sidebar at the end of this chapter.)

A DECENT INTERVAL

I'm not going to get into the particulars of Alwyn's workouts here, except to explain why he emphasizes intervals over steady-state endurance.

First, there's metabolic perturbation, which we just discussed. Since it's harder to run or ride or swim fast, it's also more inefficient. That means you shake things up more than you would at a steady pace, which leads to a bigger post-exercise response.

Second, it takes less time. You'd be hard-pressed to go longer than twenty minutes in an interval workout. Thirty minutes is a pretty good interval workout even for an advanced athlete. So you're in and out faster.

As with any type of anaerobic exercise, you force your body to use carbohydrates for energy during the high-intensity intervals. Then you use more fat when you're recovering.

You can do intervals any number of ways, with any combination of work and rest. Alwyn uses a 1:2 ratio here, so you'll go hard for a minute, say, and then rest two minutes. In his experience, that's the most effective protocol for rapid fat loss in women who aren't either elite athletes or absolute beginners. (Intervals aren't a good choice for someone who hasn't exercised since high school gym class, but I'll explain the alternatives in Chapter 11.)

Now, if you actually enjoy endurance exercise, and would miss it if you couldn't do any, we don't want to discourage you from that. But Alwyn has come up with a unique way of making it more effective.

You'll do intervals first, to work off some of the glycogen in your muscles. Then you'll step off the track or treadmill or get off the bike or out of the pool. That is, you'll stop altogether for five minutes. And then you'll get back on or in and do some steady-pace exercise at an easy pace.

Why bother? Because after you stop exercising, your body will immediately flood your bloodstream with triglycerides. Women's muscles use more of these fat molecules for energy than do men's. When you start exercising again, you'll have more fat readily available for energy, which means you'll burn more of it than you would if you'd done nothing but steady-pace work.

Does it work? Alwyn says the female clients he trains typically lose 2 pounds of fat in a week, and 6 to 10 pounds in a month. Granted, these are women whose workouts are designed and supervised by experienced and talented trainers, so we aren't promoting those numbers as the results you should expect from Alwyn's programs in *The New Rules of Lifting for Women*. And it's worth noting that the clients at Alwyn's facility are also getting nutrition advice that multiplies the effects of the training.

Which is as good an opportunity as any to move on to our diet plan.

The Heart of the Matter

Heart disease is the number-one killer of women, claiming more than 460,000 in 2004. By comparison, lung and breast cancer combined killed about 109,000. It's brought on by a combination of factors, including genetics, obesity, inactivity, and stress. There's nothing much you can do to change your genetics, but exercise is a risk modifier that's within your control, and researchers have come up with multiple ways to prescribe it for heart-disease prevention.

For example, Harvard researchers wrote in a 1999 study in the *New England Journal of Medicine* that women who walked at a brisk pace three or more hours a week were 35 percent less likely to suffer a heart attack than women who got little or no physical activity. The researchers further calculated that one and a half hours a week of "vigorous" physical activity—a category that includes jogging, serious swimming and cycling, backpacking, and sports like basketball or tennis—had about the same effect on heart-attack risk.

Other groups of researchers have tackled the question in different ways—hours spent walking, walking speed, calories burned during all types of exercise. Sometimes there's a linear relationship between amount of exercise and lowered risk of heart disease (the more you do, the lower your risk), and sometimes there's little difference between modest amounts of exercise (an hour a week, say) and a lot of it.

Two trends, though, are pretty solid:

- Some is always better than none. If "some" is all you can do, don't sweat the details.
- Harder is generally better than easier.

Scientists rate the intensity of exercise according to METs, or metabolic equivalents. The cutoff line between "moderate" and "vigorous" exercise is 6 METs, or the point at which your body is using six times as much energy as it would at rest. Serious strength training is considered a 6-MET activity, as is cross-country hiking, doubles tennis, and heavy-duty construction or landscaping work. Two hours of any of those activities in a week gives you 12 MET-hours of physical activity. According to the study I noted above, that much exercise would theoretically reduce your risk of heart disease by about 30 percent. It's the second-best of the five categories. Women in the highest category got at least 21.7 MET-hours a week of physical activity (the median was 35 MET-hours), and for their efforts were rewarded with 40 percent less heart disease than the least-active women, who got less than 1 MET-hour a week.

The most important takeaway from this research is that it's not particularly useful to think of exercise in terms of categories such as "cardio" or "weight lifting." It makes more sense to look at the total amount of exercise you get in relation to the amount of effort it takes to perform that exercise.

Below is a chart that gives you an idea of the average estimated effort involved in some popular activities. Remember that this isn't Holy Writ; two people doing the same workout, playing the same sport, or taking the same exercise class might put in different levels of effort. Even with exercises that are quantified by speed (swimming, cycling, running), one person's skill or biomechanics might be superior to another's, enabling her to swim, ride, or run more efficiently, and thus hit that pace with less effort.

Activity	METs (per hour)
Stretching / Hatha yoga	2.5*
Walking the dog	2.8
Walking 3.5 mph, level surface	3.8
Tennis (doubles)	5
Bicycling, 10–11.9 mph	6
Heavy-duty house or yard work (roofing, chopping wood, gardening with heavy equipment, shoveling snow)	6
Hiking	6
Weight lifting (working hard)	6
Backpacking	7
Skiing	7
Basketball (full-court, game conditions)	8
Beach volleyball	8
Bicycling, 12–13.9 mph	8
Rock climbing	8[†]
Running, 5 mph (12-minute miles)	8
Swimming laps (freestyle, 50 yards per minute)	8
Tennis (singles)	8
Mountain biking	8.5
Racquetball (game)	10
Running, 6.7 mph (9-minute miles)	11

* This is the only type of yoga that's been quantified in terms of METs; as of this writing, there aren't any data on Pilates or more vigorous yoga styles.

[†] On the ascent, you're at 11 METs.

PART 2

YOU AREN'T WHAT YOU DON'T EAT

The War Against Food

NEW RULE #12 • Calorie restriction is the worst idea ever

I recently visited the website of the Calorie Restriction Society, an organization that believes humans can have longer and better lives if they voluntarily limit the amount of food they consume. It's an entertainingly retro idea, like playing tennis with a wooden racquet, but the site has some deadly serious warnings about the dangers of cutting calories too quickly and too drastically. Among the horrors:

- Depression
- Loss of strength and muscle mass
- Deteriorating bone mass
- Hormonal disruption, including lower testosterone in men and amenorrhea in women
- Diminished energy and sex drive

Remember, these warnings come from a group that exists to convince people to eat less. How much less? According to one study, they eat between 1,400 and 2,000 calories a day, in a country in which people typically wolf down 2,000 to 3,000 or more a day.

Which brings me to *The Sonoma Diet,* a book that hit the *New York Times* bestseller list in early 2006.

You know how many calories the author recommends for those just starting her diet? Between 1,200 and 1,400 a day.

Yes, the *maximum* calories she allows in the first phase of her diet is equal to the *fewest* calories eaten by members of a cult who try to live longer by teetering on the precipice of starvation. This "rapid weight loss" phase is only designed to last ten days, but still, starvation is starvation. And naming a book after a beautiful place like Sonoma County, California, doesn't change that equation.

So with those scary thoughts in our minds, let's talk about calories.

THE HARD WAY

In my view, there are two fundamental approaches to weight loss: In the traditional approach, the one that advocates cutting calories, you are making two sacrifices for the goal of a smaller and leaner body:

- You're going to lose muscle mass.
- You're going to slow down your metabolism.

The metabolic slowdown has two causes. Losing muscle means you have a slower resting metabolic rate. But eating less also slows down your metabolism. About 10 percent of the calories you eat are burned off during digestion. The technical term for this is "thermic effect of food," or TEF. If you're in what's called "energy balance"— that is, you're eating and burning off the exact same number of calories over time, and not gaining or losing weight—then TEF accounts for about 10 percent of your metabolic rate. Thus, eating a lower-calorie diet decreases the TEF.

Let's run some numbers:

Say you eat 2,000 calories a day, and you're in energy balance. Call it the Goldilocks Diet—neither too many calories, nor too few. About 200 of those calories are burned off during digestion. Now let's say you decide to go on the Wicked Stepsister Diet, and you cut 500 calories a day. Aside from leaving you pretty damned hungry, you're also slowing your metabolism by about 50 calories a day. Now your TEF is about 150 calories a day, instead of 200.

On top of that, you're certainly going to lose some muscle mass. A study out of Washington University in St. Louis put a group of late-middle-aged men and women on a calorie-restricted diet for a year. They lost about 18 pounds, on average, which was about 10 percent of their body weight. (Remember, this was a mix of men and women.) They also lost 3.5 percent of their total lean mass—muscle, bone, and everything else that isn't fat—as well as 7 percent of the muscle in their thighs. Sacrificing 3.5 percent of their working parts in a year also led to decreases in strength and aerobic capacity.

I mentioned in Chapter 2 that strength is correlated with longevity in both men and women. The relationship between aerobic capacity and longevity is pretty strong, too; in a Cooper Institute study published in 2002, middle-aged women with moderate aerobic fitness were about half as likely to die of any cause as the women with the lowest fitness levels. (Curiously, the women with the highest aerobic fitness had a higher death rate than the middle group, although the rate was still 43 percent lower than that of the least-fit women.)

Put another way: A chronic low-calorie diet is a death wish, and the slowdown in metabolism is only a small part of the problem. Is there a better way? Damned glad you asked.

NEW RULE #13 • Traditional weight-loss advice is fatally flawed

Traditional weight-loss advice: "Eat less and exercise more." You've heard it more times than you can remember. I've heard it, too, but being male, I have a magical ability to filter out half the equation. I'll hear "Exercise more," and develop a strategy for that. If men like me hear "Eat less," it usually means "Eat a salad instead of a microwave burrito." And even that is usually too much dietary discipline to expect from my gender.

But let's get back to you, and take a closer look at "Eat less and exercise more." I hope I've convinced you by now that "Eat less" is a formula for slowing down your resting metabolic rate. And "Exercise more" is a way to increase your metabolic rate.

The combination, however, can be expressed this way: Slow down your metabolism while speeding it up.

Does that sound reasonable? If a financial advisor told you to run up your credit cards while putting away money in a savings account, would you take that advice? Or would you get out of his office as fast as you possibly could, employing both of your anaerobic energy systems? Would you say to your employees that you want them all to start working longer hours, and as a reward, you're going to pay them less? If you made that announcement on Friday, would anyone show up on Monday?

To put it into a political context, it's the equivalent of "I voted for it before I voted against it."

It is, to put it as simply as I can, illogical.

The reward of eating less is that you have to eat even less as you lose weight and your metabolism slows down. I don't know about you, but I can't imagine that I'd be happy if all I got out of starving myself down to a smaller waist size is that I got to experience even deeper levels of starvation.

Let's get back to that U.S. Department of Agriculture study I mentioned in Chapter 3: The women cut 50 percent of the calories from their diets, and the result was a loss of about 10 pounds of lean tissue in twelve weeks, which slowed their metabolic rates by 9 percent, which made their exercise so efficient that they burned 16 percent fewer calories while doing it at low intensities.

You wouldn't take a deal like that in any other aspect of your life, and I hope I can talk you out of accepting it as the best way to lose weight. In fact, I don't even like the phrase "weight loss." To me, it implies indiscriminate weight loss, as if it's equally beneficial to lose fat or muscle tissue, as long as the needle on the scale doesn't go as far to the right.

I like to frame it differently, and talk about "fat loss."

Now we know we're focused on the specific goal of shedding one type of weight, while preserving muscle tissue.

NEW RULE #14 • To reach your goals, you may need to eat more

I understand no one bought this book to learn to eat more. Every one of us already knows how to do that. But what I'm talking about is eating more in strategic circumstances. Some call it "nutrition timing." Just about everybody in the body-transformation biz uses it with their clients, and of course they do it for themselves.

The idea is simple: If you time your meals to coincide with your workouts, you enhance the muscle-building effects of those workouts. (I'll discuss this in more detail in chapters 6 and 7.) But coordinating fitness and food also increases the TEF of those meals. A small study at the University of Nevada Las Vegas found that subjects burned off 73 percent more calories when a meal followed a strength-training session. Six of the nine subjects in the study were women. Another study, from the University of Colorado, found that habitual exercisers have a 25 percent higher TEF than nonexercisers. The subjects in the latter study were all men, but it shouldn't matter; other research from that same group has shown there isn't a gender difference in TEF.

All that said, the best way to illustrate the importance of eating enough calories is to take a closer look at what goes wrong when you don't.

WHEN HORMONES ATTACK

As I was writing this chapter, in December 2006, a study came out showing that underweight women who became pregnant were 72 percent more likely to have a miscarriage. "Underweight" was described as a body mass index (BMI) of 18.5 or less. To give you a reference point, a woman who is five-foot-four and weighs 107 pounds would have a BMI of 18.4, and would thus be considered underweight in this study.

Two things jumped out at me as I read that:

First, I'd guess that most of the women we see on TV and in the movies fall into the "underweight" category. So the role models you grew up with, and our daughters will grow up with, are at an unhealthy weight, never mind unrealistic for most who'd try to achieve it.

Second, it doesn't surprise me at all to learn that a low body weight—usually achieved with a low-calorie diet—would interrupt reproductive function. A woman's reproductive hormones are highly sensitive to nutrition, for a simple evolutionary reason: It makes no sense to get pregnant during periods in which starvation is a distinct possibility. So your body shifts its priorities elsewhere, fueling your brain and internal organs rather than allocating those precious energy reserves to a hungry offspring. For most of human history, being pregnant and then delivering a child in times of famine gives the family two distinct disadvantages: not only is the family risking the loss of the fetus, but the mother's health would be compromised as well.

I bring up reproductive function, and reproductive hormones, because they're a very good stand-in for your general health. If you're premenopausal and your estrogen is low—as it would be if you're not eating enough—you're not going to build the healthy reserves of bone tissue that you'll need when you're postmenopausal and your bones start shrinking from lack of estrogen.

And it's not just the reproductive hormones; if you're starving yourself to achieve a photogenic level of emaciation, you're also disrupting chemicals that, ironically, keep your metabolism up and help you control your weight. These disruptions help explain why rapid-weight-loss diets are such a metabolic disaster. When you start re-gaining weight—and you always will, since self-starvation is impossible to maintain for most of us—a much higher percentage will appear on your body in the form of fat, rather than the normal mix of fat and lean tissue.

Let's start with estrogen.

In sports medicine, it's well established that female athletes who train hard and don't get enough calories will experience amenorrhea. That is, they'll stop having periods—a clear sign of low estrogen levels. More recently, it's been shown that female athletes with low estrogen levels will have more stress fractures. As they go through life, the loss of bone minerals will continue to haunt them, leading to much more se-rious fractures in old age.

Studies by Anne Loucks, Ph.D., have shown that exercise isn't the sole culprit; it's the lack of calories combined with serious exercise that lowers estrogen levels.

Amenorrhea is an obvious symptom of undereating. When you go a couple months without a period, you know something's wrong. But most of the conse-quences of undereating aren't immediately obvious. Among the hormones that could go haywire:

Luteinizing hormone, which is responsible for triggering ovulation.

Leptin, which regulates appetite and metabolism (less leptin means more hunger, and less satiety from the food you eat).

Thyroid hormones, which control not only your resting metabolic rate, but also the metabolism of protein, carbohydrates, and fat. One kinda-sorta good way to tell if you have low thyroid-hormone levels is if you notice you feel cold after eating. These hormones decline in hibernating mammals, whose body temperature falls rap-idly when it's time to sack out for the winter. So if your levels are low, your body might feel as if it's going into hibernation after a meal.

Cortisol, a stress hormone, rises when you're chronically undernourished, and it's about the last hormone you want more of. Cortisol strips your muscles of protein and turns it into sugar for energy. That's why cortisol is also linked to higher blood sugar, as well as higher blood pressure and suppression of your immune system.

The net result of these hormones getting all medieval on you is what I've harped on throughout this chapter: Your resting metabolic rate slows. You're voting for a leaner body by working out, but you're voting against it by eating too little food.

The Carb Wars Are So Over

WE LIVE IN an age in which the phrase "refined carbs" has the same dreaded resonance as "we've found irregularities in your expense report." Still, you don't have to look far to find women who still believe "fat makes you fat." A corollary belief is that dietary protein is somehow unsavory—you know there must be something wrong with a protein-rich diet if people like the late Dr. Atkins were in favor and all the esteemed experts of nutrition science were opposed.

So if carbs are satanic, fat makes you fat, and protein is the province of people you've been told not to trust, that leaves us with a steady diet of . . . water. (In case you're wondering, I'm not going to say anything negative about water. It would make for a more entertaining book, but it would also be difficult to do with a straight face.)

Let's relax, take a deep breath, and think all this through. First off, it's worth remembering that humans are the original hybrid vehicles. Our bodies can run on anything. I mentioned in Chapter 3 that we prefer to burn a mix of carbohydrate (in the form of glycogen, or blood sugar) and fat throughout the day. But that doesn't mean you actually have to eat a balance of carbs and fat. Your body can make triglycerides, the form of fat it uses for energy, from carbohydrates. Or it can make glycogen from fat. And if you somehow managed to eat pure protein without any carbs or fat, your body could turn that into several different forms of energy as well.

My point is that your body is astoundingly adaptable. Because it's designed for survival in many different climates, with many different forms of sustenance, you could eat just about anything that falls into the general category of "food" and live to tell the story to your grandchildren, assuming you don't have to eat that suboptimal diet for long.

Here's an example of how flexible your body is:

Your brain is just 2 percent of your total body weight, but sucks up fully 20 percent of your daily calorie expenditure. (Sort of makes you want to use it more productively, doesn't it?) And, despite the fact your brain is made mostly of fat, it runs entirely on sugar. But that doesn't mean you have to eat 20 percent of your calories in the form of carbohydrates. You could eat more, or you could eat less, and your brain would still work.

Which brings me to the concept of macronutrient ratios. Don't get put off by the jargon. Yeah, I know, I say that a lot, but this time I really mean it. There are only three macronutrients: carbohydrate, protein, and fat. Everything else is water, ash, or alcohol, the last of which doesn't fall neatly into the other categories. It's technically a carbohydrate but has some fat-like qualities. (If you're ingesting enough alcohol for this to be an issue, I suggest you rethink that strategy.) I have good reason to burden you with the eight syllables of "macronutrient ratio." Since *The Zone* came out in 1995, we've had a fascination with the idea that there's an ideal combination of the three macronutrients, a ratio that will work for all people, all the time.

Is there such a thing? Let's discuss.

NEW RULE #15 • On balance, a balanced macro diet is best

I entered the carb wars with my first book, *The Testosterone Advantage Plan*, published in 2002. The diet my coauthors and I recommended emphasized protein and healthy fats and said some discouraging words about carbohydrates. Still, between one-third and two-fifths of the calories in the diet came from carbs—primarily fruits, vegetables, beans, and whole grains, along with the carbs in nuts and dairy products.

The book wasn't controversial at all in the outside world, six years after *The Zone* had immortalized "40/30/30," its recommended combination of 40 percent carbohydrate, 30 percent fat, and 30 percent protein. That was more or less what we recommended, although we couldn't think of any reason why anyone had to hit this ratio with every single meal, as *The Zone* required. But inside the company I worked for at the time, you'd have thought we were telling readers to eat sticks of butter dipped in Crisco. Colleagues of mine were lobbying our bosses to kill the book.

They lost that battle, but won in the end. Our own company published the low-carb *South Beach Diet* in the spring of 2003, and everyone forgot *Testosterone Advantage Plan* even existed.

SBD, which came out the same week that Dr. Robert Atkins slipped on a patch of ice and suffered a fatal brain injury, put a friendlier face on the advice to avoid carbs—call it "compassionate carbophobia." Its flexibility also helped diet-conscious readers back away from their Zone-inspired obsession with macronutrient ratios.

Ironically, this change came just as nutritional science was inching toward an unspoken consensus on the ideal combination of carbs, fat, and protein.

Most intriguing to me was a study from Tufts–New England Medical Center published in 2005. It compared four popular diet plans—Atkins, Zone, Weight Watchers, Ornish—by placing actual people on them for a year. But the study wasn't just about weight loss; if it had been, the super-low-fat Ornish diet would've been judged the best. (There was little difference in weight loss across the board; the "best" and "worst" of the four were separated by less than 3 pounds of weight lost in twelve months.) It also looked at adherence—who stuck with each diet. The adherence winners were Zone and Weight Watchers; 65 percent of the participants in each group followed the diet for a year. Ornish came in last, with just 50 percent adherence versus 53 percent for Atkins.

I came away with the idea that none of the diets worked particularly well.

But that's not really fair to any of them. There's a huge difference between Ornish and Atkins, and a lesser but still important distinction between Weight Watchers and the Zone. Weight Watchers is agnostic on the subject of macronutrients—all foods are assigned points based on a variety of factors, and you can eat them in whatever combination you choose, as long as you stick to a set point total per day. The Zone, meanwhile, fetishizes the importance of hitting the right combination every time you eat.

So why didn't those differences matter, in terms of weight loss? My guess: because people are as different as the four diets. In the real world, nobody is randomly assigned to a diet as extreme as Atkins or Ornish. That only happens in scientific research. If you choose to go to those lengths to lose weight or improve your health, it's something you inflict upon yourself. Had someone randomly assigned me to the Ornish plan, I'd have dropped out the first week. And if someone who wanted to try a low-fat diet got stuck in the Atkins group, I'd expect a similar reaction.

No study is perfect, though, and most of the ones I've seen show at least a bit of bias in their design. A study that plays it straight with four very different and potentially controversial diets is to be admired, and to be taken seriously. And if we take this study seriously, we see that the Zone diet comes out best, by a nose. It was tied for the best adherence, and offered the second-best weight loss.

You can find support for the idea of balancing macronutrients just about anywhere you look. Studies that compare higher-protein plans with lower-protein plans almost always show that the protein makes a difference. (I say "almost always" because no conclusion holds in every single published study.) That is, the diet plan with more protein usually comes out ahead.

The magic number seems to be about 30 percent of total calories. That's twice the amount of protein you'll find in a typical American diet, but it's a feature in the Zone, Atkins, and South Beach diets. A variety of studies and reviews suggest that if 30 percent of your daily calories come from protein, you'll end up eating fewer total calories, since protein is more satiating, leaving you feeling fuller longer between meals. You'll also probably weigh less, since protein requires a lot more energy to digest than any other macronutrient. (This is the thermic effect of feeding, TEF, which we covered in Chapter 4.)

NEW RULE #16 • Protein is the queen of macronutrients

Protein does more than blunt your appetite and speed up your metabolism. It also helps you maintain muscle while losing fat. For example, a University of Illinois study published in 2005 took a group of middle-aged women and split them into four groups. Two groups had higher-protein diets with few carbs, and two ate lower-protein meals with higher carbs. One group from each side exercised (a combination of strength training and walking), while the others just changed their diets without exercising. The protein-plus-exercise group lost the most weight (22 pounds, on average), and retained all but 1 pound of their muscle mass. Conversely, the carbs-plus-exercise group lost an average of 15 pounds, which included 2 pounds of muscle. Even more remarkable was that the higher-protein exercisers lost 11 pounds of middle-body fat versus 7 pounds for their carb-eating counterparts.

Higher-protein diets seem to work regardless of the relative amounts of fat and carbohydrate. I've seen higher protein produce better results in high-fat and low-fat diets, and in diets relatively high or low in carbs. Protein is to diets what black is to fashion: it makes everyone thinner.

That leaves us in a position to choose our own combination of carbs and fat. It's safe to say that some amount of each is important. Since fats are crucial for the development and proper function of your hormones, and since your body can't make certain types of fats and thus needs to get them from your diet, a low-fat approach makes little sense.

Conversely, I don't think a low-carb approach would be in your best interest, either, unless you have diabetes or a specific medical condition that requires such a diet. Alwyn's workouts require a lot of energy, pulling glucose from your blood and glycogen from your muscles at the same time you're deliberately inducing damage in your muscle fibers and connective tissues. You need to replace that glycogen in your muscles, just as you need to give your body protein to repair your working parts. You could accomplish both goals with a low-carb diet, but it's not the easiest, most direct, or most convenient way to do it.

I'm deliberately hedging with my language here, because there simply is no settled approach that works for everybody. If I were your doctor and knew you were diabetic, of course I'd give you a low-carb plan, and concede that your muscles will have to make do without a large and constant supply of readily accessible sugar. If you were extremely overweight, I'd probably make the same recommendation. But if there were a compelling reason to design a low-fat and/or low-protein plan (kidney disease, for example), we could do that as well. But in the absence of any specific and urgent reason to limit carbs or fat, the path of least resistance leads to balanced macronutrients. Once you brush aside ideology, the balanced-macro strategy ensures you get plenty of everything without too much of anything.

Allow me one last argument:

My friend Susan Kleiner, R.D., Ph.D., is a sports nutritionist in Seattle who works with elite athletes at every level, along with nonathletes. She's always been someone who combined current science with the most practical applications to get the best results for her clients. I've never heard her proselytize for any particular dietary philosophy. Her latest book is called *The Good Mood Diet*, and in it she recommends a specific macronutrient ratio: 40/30/30. I asked her why she did that, and why she chose the one she did.

"A diet with less than 40 percent carbs is depressing—literally. Forty percent is also better for fat loss," she told me. "A diet with less than 25 to 30 percent fat lowers coping skills and raises anxiety, anger, and hostility levels." She went on to explain how she ended up at 30 percent protein, which turns out to be roughly the same calculation we use—2 grams of protein per kilogram (2.2 pounds) of body weight per day comes out to about 30 percent of calories for a typical woman eating the typical amount of food we recommend. Protein improves mood because of tryptophan, an amino acid you've probably heard of. (It played a role in a memorable episode of *Seinfeld*. Jerry, Elaine, and George feed tryptophan-rich turkey breast to one of Jerry's girlfriends so she'll doze off and they can play with the vintage toys she's collected but won't let any of them touch when she's awake.)

To sum up, the bottom line on macronutrients is really a lot more straightforward than many nutrition experts make it seem. You need some of each, and given the fact we modern humans have the luxury to choose our own proportions, the best choice is a roughly equal mix. Too much of one thing means too little of something else, and each imbalance presents its own set of problems.

But the most underrated reason for choosing balance is the one that probably matters most for long-term success: It's easier.

So that's how we came up with the structure of the meal plan. In the next chapter, I'll talk about the specifics.

Good Nutrition: Simple Versus Simplistic

IF EVERYTHING my coauthors and I recommend were to be summed up in three steps, it's hard to go wrong with these:

- Metabolism
- Anerobic exercise
- Nutritional consistency

Conveniently, they give us a nice, easy-to-remember acronym—MAN (as in Lift Like a . . .).

I've talked already about the importance of maintaining or even increasing your metabolic rate; it's the key to weight control without a lifetime of deprivation.

And you know how I feel about anaerobic exercise. A base of endurance is important—if you can't walk at a brisk pace for a half-hour without stopping for defibrillation, or ride a bike for a couple hours at a leisurely pace with your friends . . . well, you need to fix that. The human body, as I've said, is designed to walk long distances on foot, and if you can't even manage relatively short distances, you're in trouble.

So I'm not by any means disparaging the need for some endurance capability. My goal is to promote anaerobic exercise as not only the ticket to a better body now—the subject of this book, if that's not clear—but also the key to lifelong strength and mobility. You don't want to get to the point where you can't get out of a chair unassisted, or walk up a flight of stairs, or do a short little hop over some puddle of nastiness on the sidewalk. I know it seems absurd to worry about those things now, but when you're eighty or ninety, anaerobic fitness will be the difference between a nursing home and that worldwide cruise you can finally afford.

This chapter is about the N: nutritional consistency. Once you separate nutrition science and practice from the preconceived notions that often drive them, what you're left with is the need to be nutritionally consistent—to eat the best foods, avoid the worst ones, practice moderation, avoid long stretches without any food at all, and, most of all, to employ all these habits almost all the time.

It's easier than you think, once you know the basics.

NEW RULE #17 • More meals are better than fewer

Smart people like to debate the question of how many daily meals or snacks is best. In our plan, we advocate five or six a day—three traditional meals and two or three snacks, or mini-meals. (You'll get to six on the days you work out, since you'll have a post-workout shake; other days have five.) Our goals:

- You want to ensure you have enough food in your system, and that you get it frequently enough. It's important to avoid the hunger pangs that screw up even the best diet plans.
- Frequent eating reminds you that you're on a quest to improve your health and physique. This is subjective (a hunch, in other words), but I suspect that it's easier to stay with the program if you have to act on it five or six times a day versus three or four. The more times a day you remind yourself to eat the foods that will help you succeed, the less chance there is that you'll slip up.
- There is a mild metabolic benefit to eating frequently and regularly.

The last bullet point comes from a small English study published in 2004. The women in the study were tested after eating a steady pattern of six meals a day versus varying patterns of three to nine daily meals. What the researchers found is that the women had a lower thermic effect of feeding—TEF—when they varied their meal pattern day after day. Or, to put it another way, they burned more calories after meals when they followed a steady pattern of six meals a day.

An artificial setup? Sure. I've never met anyone who jumped from three to nine meals a day and back again. But it does show that there's a real physiological effect of choosing one consistent pattern.

That leads to a logical question: Does the number of meals matter, as long as there's a consistent pattern? In other words, would three meals a day work as well as four, five, or six?

An article by a group of French researchers, published in the Swiss Forum of Nutrition series, sheds a bit of light on that question. In France, most children and many adults eat a fourth daily meal in between lunch and dinner. When researchers looked at adults who were accustomed to eating that fourth meal, but then stopped, they found that the meal-skippers were heavier than a comparable group who kept eating the fourth meal. But here's the kicker: *Both groups ate the same number of calories.* The group who spread those calories over four meals weighed less than those who squeezed them into three.

A lot of nutritionists today will still tell you that the only determinant of your weight is calories in and calories out—how much you eat and how much you burn off. But here you have people who ate the same amount of food, but ate it differently, and gained weight.

If nothing else, these two studies make a strong argument for establishing a pattern and sticking with it.

Let's get back to TEF, the subject of the first study. Back in 1998, an Italian study showed that the higher the TEF of a meal, the more satiety you enjoy afterward—you feel full longer between meals. It's sort of a "duh!" conclusion, given that we know protein creates a much higher TEF than fat or carbohydrate, and that protein also leads to greater satiety. So it's easy enough to say, "Eat more protein at every meal."

But if TEF itself—the calories you're burning after a meal—contributes to satiety, and that effect might be independent of the type of food you're eating, then we have another solid reason to stick with a consistent meal pattern. And we also have a reason to eat something immediately after a workout. As I showed in Chapter 4, the TEF is much higher for food eaten in that window of opportunity.

Put it all together, and I think there's a solid case for a consistent pattern of eating at least four times a day. Moreover, I can't see any reason to stop with four. If you go up to five, you can have a snack (or mini-meal, or whatever you prefer to call it) between breakfast and lunch, along with the one between lunch and dinner. Then, on the days you lift weights, you'll eat six times, including the protein shake you have as soon as possible after your workout. If you do that consistently—and believe me, it's easier than it sounds—you should get every possible metabolic benefit from your meal plan.

FAT OUT OF HELL

I have bad days, when I think everything I've advocated about fitness and nutrition has led to the opposite behavior. One of the darkest of those dark days came when I saw a "Low Fat!" banner on a package of candy. I'm not disputing the accuracy—*of course* a product that's mostly sugar won't have much fat—but I resent the implication that candy is good for you by virtue of the fact it's not butter. In fact, I'd probably argue that in some circumstances butter is better for you than candy, calorie for calorie. At least your body can use some of the fats in butter to produce hormones and shore up your body's structures at the cellular level. Sugar is a one-trick pony. It provides energy, and that's it. As I said in Chapter 5, you can use just about anything digestible for energy, including butter. Heck, maybe we'll see the day when the National Dairy Council will promote butter as "sugar-free."

Before I get into the specific types of fat, and the advantages and disadvantages of each, let's cast a wider net and ask the most obvious question: Is there any inherent danger in eating fat of any type, in any quantity?

The Nurses' Health Study, an ongoing look at the health of some 80,000 women being tracked by Harvard Medical School researchers, tried to answer the big "fat" question by looking at the relationship between dietary fat and heart disease. If the question is, "Is it better to eat more fat, or less?" the answer is, "You're asking the wrong question." There isn't an overall trend, once you adjust for everything—family history, lifestyle, body weight, consumption of other types of foods, and so on. (It's also worth noting that few women in the study actually follow a low-fat diet.)

The researchers drew two main conclusions:

- To no one's surprise, the study showed that those eating the most trans fats had the most heart disease. You already knew that trans fats—those that start as one type of fat but are altered to make them more stable for cooking, using a process called hydrogenation—are to be avoided.
- Women eating the most polyunsaturated fats had a one-third reduction in heart-disease risk, compared to women who ate the least.

Which sounds great . . . except it doesn't mean a thing until you understand the distinctions between different types of unsaturated fats. There's no simple way to tell. Labels tell us how much total fat, saturated fat, and trans fat you'll find in any given food (assuming it's a food that comes in a package, which rules out fresh meat, fish, and produce). But they don't say how much unsaturated fat a food contains, or what type. So here's a quick primer on the different types, where you're most likely to find them, and what each does for your body:

Monounsaturated fat

These are the fats that are most prevalent in olive oil, avocados, and nuts. About half the fats in peanuts, chicken, and various meats are monounsaturated. These fats are "nonessential," which means your body can make them from other fats you eat. They're also considered beneficial, meaning they don't present any negative consequences (they don't change your cholesterol levels, for example), and they're easy to use for energy and to make hormones.

About nuts, which are great sources of monounsaturated fats:

I mentioned the Nurses' Health Study a few paragraphs ago. (And I'll mention it again a few paragraphs ahead.) Another paper that came out of that ongoing project looked at low-carb diets. The object was to see whether, as doctors and nutritionists have long warned, such diets would lead to more heart disease. The short answer is no, but buried in the data was something really interesting: The group with the lowest heart-disease risk—about 30 percent below baseline—were those who ate the most nuts. They averaged 2.8 servings of nuts per week, which was a lot more than any other group in the study ate. Since a serving is about a quarter cup, you should get some cardiac protection with just three-quarters of a cup of nuts a week.

Omega-6 polyunsaturated fat

This is one of the main categories of polyunsaturated fats, and by far the most common. You find it in meat, fish, eggs, nuts, and many kinds of oils. Vegetable oils are the biggest source of omega-6 polys in our diets; they're especially rich in a type of omega-6 called linoleic acid.

Don't feel any pressure to remember the names of individual fatty acids, because I sure don't. I have to look them up every time I write about fat in an article or book. I mention linoleic acid for two reasons:

- It's the single most prevalent omega-6 fat in our diets, since it's found in most prepared foods that use vegetable oil. Soybean oil, for example, is the main ingredient in mayonnaise and salad dressing, and is the single greatest contributor of linoleic acid to our diets.
- It's the only fat in the Nurses' Health Study that was associated with a steady decline in heart-disease risk with increased consumption. The more you eat, the less risk you have.

I'll confess I find it tough to get my brain around the idea of mayonnaise as a health food. Fortunately for my sanity, it's not. Omega-6 fats in general and linoleic acid in particular have been linked to both breast and prostate cancer, and that may not be the worst damage they do. When pregnant and nursing mothers consume high amounts of linoleic acid, their children are more likely to be obese.

Still, I'm surprised it has the opposite effect when it comes to heart-attack risk. My guess is that this is because of the fat's well-known ability to lower your level of LDL, the "bad" cholesterol.

That said, there seems to be an upper limit to how much linoleic acid you can eat before its benefits are negated—probably about 10 percent of the total calories in your diet. So if you eat 2,000 calories a day, the most linoleic acid you could safely eat would be 200 calories' worth, or about 18 grams. (Fat has 9 calories per gram.) Since you'll never find pure linoleic acid in any foods you eat—even soybean oil gets just half its calories from omega-6 fats, not all of which are linoleic acid—it's unlikely you'll pass that limit.

But if you do, the health risks are sobering. You're more likely to get gallstones, and less likely to realize the benefits of HDL, the "good" cholesterol. Your fat cells will be more vulnerable to damage from rogue molecules called free radicals, which can lead to premature aging, at best, or cancer, as aforementioned, at worst.

Too much linoleic acid can also disrupt the actions of omega-3 fats, which, as you'll read, are probably the healthiest of all.

Omega-3 polyunsaturated fat

This type of fat has been associated with better heart health, a faster metabolism, stronger joints, lower rates of depression, and just about every beneficial outcome short of helping you pay off your credit-card balance. Omega-3 fats are especially crucial in the first few months of life, spurring the development of an infant's brain, eyesight, and overall growth.

Like omega-6 fat, it's considered "essential," which means it must come from your diet. That can be a problem. Humans evolved with abundant omega-3 fats in the food chain. Wild grasses had lots of these fats (and still do), and animals that grazed on them stored that fat. So when one of our ancient ancestors had a chunk of mastodon or wooly rhino for lunch, she was getting more omega-3 fat than we get from the meat we buy in stores today. (For that matter, our grandparents probably ate more grass-fed beef than we do.) Animals in our modern system have been fed corn, instead of grass, so the polyunsaturated fats in their meats will tend to be rich in omega-6 fats and relatively sparse in omega-3s.

The best sources of omega-3 fat in our diets today are fish and fish oil. It's also found in canola oil, flaxseed and flaxseed oil, and walnuts. Cassandra has included some fish in our meal plans, and recommends fish oil supplements. (I take several fish-oil capsules a day, as do most of the people I talk to in the fitness business.)

In the previous section I noted that omega-6 fats have been linked to the growth of cancer cells. Interestingly, omega-3 fats do the opposite—they seem to shrink those cells. Researchers have speculated that humans evolved to eat omega-6 and omega-3 fats in relatively equal proportions, but the modern food chain has taken out most of the latter while dramatically increasing the former.

Another way to get more omega-3s in your diet is to go out of your way to purchase meat, eggs, and dairy products from animals that have been allowed to graze in pastures, rather than kept in confined spaces and fed corn and other grains. Milk and cheese from pasture-raised cattle will also be higher in a type of fat called CLA, which is short for conjugated linoleic acid. If I were good at chemistry (I barely passed my only high-school class in the subject) I might have a fighting chance of understanding why the slight structural difference between linoleic acid and conjugated linoleic acid makes the latter one of the healthiest fats in our food chain. CLA not only has cancer-stopping properties, it's been shown to be a potent fat-fighter in animal studies. It appears to do that in two different ways: First, it increases metabolism. Second, it increases "excreta"—which is how researchers say "It goes in one end and out the other" without resorting to bathroom jokes.

There's one more type of fat worth discussing:

Saturated fat

The safe path here is to say, "Saturated fat is bad. Eat as little as possible." The path of most resistance would be to justify eating more of it. But the most interesting trail to follow leads to the conclusion that it's not nearly as dangerous as it's been made out to be . . . which doesn't mean it's a particularly good source of daily calories, or something you should seek more of. It just means that the amounts you typically eat aren't dangerous to your health.

Generally speaking, saturated fats are those that are solid at room temperature but aren't trans fats. (You find them most often in animal products, along with coconut, palm, and peanut oils.) The Nurses' Health Study found no dangers from saturated fats, once everything else was balanced out. That may strike you as a broad caveat, but I think the take-home message is that people who have lots of unhealthy habits probably eat more saturated fat than people who try to live clean, moderate, well-balanced lives. People who actually pay attention to nutrition advice are less likely to eat the fattiest steaks, just as they're more likely to exercise, get plenty of sleep, and eat their vegetables.

Which leads me to a similarly broad conclusion about diet and exercise: basically, all health-conscious people end up at the same place. They all live longer and have fewer disabilities than people who let themselves go. The particulars aren't as important as the fundamental choice to exercise, eat well, and enjoy life without overdoing it.

Example:

A study published in 2006 reviewed research on people who eat vegetarian and vegan diets, and then compared those findings with data from similar studies of health-conscious people who aren't vegetarians. The researchers found that the vegetarians ate more of the good things you'd expect vegetarians to eat, as well as less protein, saturated fat, and omega-3 fat than the rest of us. The vegans also got by with less calcium, and as a group the non-meat-eaters tended to weigh less and have lower cholesterol levels than healthy omnivores. Their death rates from heart disease were lower, which isn't a surprise, and is clearly an important benefit. About 38 percent of women's deaths in the United States are from heart disease.

But both groups—vegetarians and meat-eaters—had about the same rates of cancer and all-cause mortality. In other words, even though the vegetarians had lower heart-disease rates, they didn't live longer than omnivores. So if you're most worried about heart disease, perhaps because of your family's medical history, then eating more vegetables and fewer foods containing saturated fat might be a good idea. But if your health concerns are more general, and you're just looking to be active and healthy for as long as possible, then there's no clear advantage to a vegetarian or vegan diet.

There are many aspects of health and nutrition to worry about; a little saturated fat isn't one of them.

CARB BLANCHE

I remember the first time I heard about *Body for Life.* I reviewed health and fitness books for Amazon.com back then, and my editor there called me up with an urgent request. The book was already Amazon's number-one best seller, a full month before its scheduled publication in June 1999, and the website needed a review, pronto. One part of the book, which I noted in my review, stuck in my mind: for reasons I couldn't fathom at the time, author Bill Phillips made a distinction between "carbohydrates" and "vegetables."

I get it now. At the time Phillips was writing *BFL,* the prevalent idea was that all carbs were good for you and all fat was bad. Vegetables and Wonder Bread were all crammed into the virtuous category of "complex carbohydrates." Phillips was trying to make the point that a lot of people he knew were getting fatter from doing what they thought they were supposed to do—eating less fat, and more carbs.

But no one was getting fat from eating vegetables, which, because of their fiber content, are as close as you can get to "free" calories. Odds are that the more of them you eat, the less you'll weigh.

I bring up a book published in 1999 for a reason. As I was writing this chapter, in the closing weeks of 2006, a health column in *The Washington Post* quoted an expert who said, yes, that consumers were completely confused about carbohydrates. "In the abstract . . . people think carbohydrates mean bread and pasta. So a lot of people are shocked when I say that fruit and vegetables are carbohydrates."

That doesn't mean anybody's confused about the benefits of fruits and vegetables, which are so abundant and obvious that they aren't worth reviewing here. It just means most of us are bogged down in definitions.

Which, I'll concede, is understandable. That's why I want you to learn the phrase "macronutrient ratios." If you want to understand what you're eating, and why, you have to start with the general categories and work your way down to the specifics. Most of us go the other direction—we know all kinds of specifics, but are vague on the big picture.

For example, you know you're supposed to eat complex carbohydrates and avoid simple carbs. So if I put an apple and a slice of angel food cake in front of you and told you it was okay to eat the simple carbs, how long would it take you to get that angel food cake into your stomach? Heck, you wouldn't even bother chewing. But you'd flunk the test. Grains are complex carbs and fruits are simple ones, so even a dessert made from highly refined flour is still an example of complex carbohydrates. And that totally virtuous apple? Simple carbs.

You should conclude, correctly, that some of the terminology you have stuck in your head is utterly meaningless. The carbs in apples and Skittles are simple. Those in cupcakes and long-grain wild rice are complex. So let's start this discussion of carbs with the idea that we'll only discuss what matters. "Simple" versus "complex" doesn't make the cut.

I also won't even try to rank carb-rich foods according to calories or vitamin content or which thing has more phyto-orgasmanutrients than the next thing. My only goal in this section is to compare foods to each other within their own categories, and provide you with a few guidelines for making the best choices when you shop or dine out. As I said, the details don't really matter until you have a grasp of the big picture.

Fruits and vegetables

You've probably heard the advice to seek out a variety of colors: blue and purple (berries and eggplant), red (strawberries and tomatoes), yellow/orange (bananas, cantaloupe, carrots, pumpkin), and green (kiwi, broccoli, and just about every type of lettuce).

If you're a regular reader of newspapers and magazines, you've probably seen lists that attempt to sort these out by the quality and quantity of vitamins and minerals. That's all interesting to know, but if you want to make it easier on yourself, you can simply pick the fruits and vegetables with the deepest colors.

So you'd pick spinach over iceberg lettuce (no surprise), and cantaloupe over bananas. A medium banana has about 100 calories, with just 3 grams of fiber and a bit of vitamin C. But if you ate half of a medium-size cantaloupe instead, you'd get about the same amount of fiber with fewer calories. You'd also get close to ten times the amount of vitamin C found in a banana, and a lot of vitamin A.

Sometimes the darkest vegetable is the least appealing (yeah, beets, I'm talkin' to you), just as the deepest leafy green (kale, perhaps) could be the most difficult to prepare.

Still, it's hard to go wrong using these two criteria: color, and the deepness and richness of the color.

Potatoes are a different type of vegetable. Unlike most of the others on this list, they're high in starch, a complex carbohydrate that converts quickly to glucose during digestion, providing fast but unsustainable energy—a drive-by on your bloodstream. (The grains discussed in the next section also contain starch as their primary carbohydrate.)

Now, the presence of starch doesn't, by itself, make the food a poor choice. Sweet potatoes, for example, are filled with carotenoids, a class of nutrients that convert to vitamin A, an antioxidant and all-around disease fighter.

White potatoes have fewer nutrients and hit your bloodstream much, much faster than sweet potatoes, due to their low fiber content and high concentration of starches. If you're going to have white potatoes, or any faster-acting starches, eat them in the first meal after a workout. That's the one time of day when you want the carbohydrates to get into your bloodstream ASAP. And here's a fun fact I learned from Cassandra while writing this chapter: Your body digests warm starches faster than cool ones. So a cold potato or slice of cold pizza provides a slower and steadier supply of energy than either would fresh from the oven. Who would've guessed that?

Grains

This is an easy category to navigate. You can divide grains into two categories:

* whole
* refined

Whole grains should have more fiber and protein than refined grains, which means they're slower to digest. The list of health benefits associated with whole grains is long and growing: better weight control, less heart disease, less cancer, lower risk of diabetes. It's impossible to say if those benefits accrue from the fiber, the protein, the disease-fighting antioxidants, or some combination. But I think I can say, with no risk of a health scientist challenging me to a duel, that without their natural fiber, protein, and antioxidants, grains offer nothing besides calories.

That's exactly what you get when you have refined grains. They're processed to improve their flavor, and the result is breads and pastas and breakfast cereals with no nutritional virtue. Manufacturers know this, which is why they often label refined grains as "enriched," which really means the opposite of enriched. After the useful nutrients have been lost in the quest for palatability, manufacturers add in a bunch of vitamins and minerals.

I don't mean to imply that all processing is bad. We don't really have anything in our food supply that isn't processed, fertilized, cross-bred, hormonally enhanced, and/or genetically manipulated. Whole grains, at least, give us food that's *minimally* processed. Another way to say that:

Whole grains leave more of the original structure of the food intact.

Processed grains, even those "enriched" with vitamins and minerals, have nothing to slow down their trek to your bloodstream. People who eat lots of processed grains and few whole grains tend to have higher levels of insulin and blood sugar, which, as you probably know, are the harbingers of diabetes and heart disease.

Wheat is by far the most popular grain in the American food supply, accounting for between two-thirds and three-quarters of total grain consumption, followed by rice and corn (although I'd guess that most Americans consider corn to be a vegetable, rather than a grain). Less common are oats, bulgur, quinoa, and couscous. More and more, products featuring the whole-grain versions of these foods advertise it prominently on the packaging. Just a cursory look through my kitchen cabinets turned up whole-grain boasts on everything from breakfast cereal to brown rice to microwave popcorn.

In other words, you won't have any trouble finding the whole-grain products in your grocery store. Even if the package doesn't make the claim as a selling point, you can look at the list of ingredients. The first ingredient should be described with the words "whole wheat" or "whole grain."

I guess it's possible that some products won't advertise their biggest selling point. Some pointers:

- Brown rice is a whole-grain product; white rice isn't. Long-grain rice can be either whole or refined, depending on whether it's brown or white. (Wild rice, by the way, is a seed, rather than a grain.)
- With oatmeal, look for either "large-flake" or "old-fashioned."

When reading labels, don't stop with the first ingredient. Lots of breakfast cereals have added sugar ("high-fructose corn syrup" is a sugar, one that's cheaper and potentially worse for you than traditional sweeteners made from sugarcane), as do whole-wheat breads and instant, microwavable oatmeal.

If you're comparing two or more products and can't tell which is better from the ingredients listed on their labels, here's a simple tiebreaker you can use: Which product has the most fiber and/or protein? That should tell you which is the least processed. A good benchmark is 4 grams of fiber per serving. That product will most likely have fewer calories per serving as well.

Beans

I know I'm supposed to call this category of carbs legumes, but you can't possibly say that word without sounding like a dork. I'm embarrassed to even type it. What we're talking about here is a class of foods that includes black and brown beans, green peas, chickpeas (also called garbanzos), navy beans, string beans, lima beans, lentils, and I don't know how many others. Peanuts are technically beans, but because they're so rich in monounsaturated fat, are usually lumped in with seeds and nuts.

Beans are the best sources of fiber in the world, and a great source of vegetable protein. The combination makes them digest about as slowly as any carbohydrates you'll find. They also tend to be low in fat, with the exception of peanuts (which are also anomalously low in fiber).

There's virtually no drawback to eating beans, aside from digestive issues. (If you're starting with dried beans, soak them for a while and then rinse them, and repeat once or twice.) You don't want to eat something with this much fiber shortly before a workout, since the exercise would interfere with digestion, and the digestion would interfere with the exercise. But any other time of day, it's hard to go wrong.

MUSCLE CHOW

I talked about protein in chapters 4 and 5—obliquely, in the discussion of the thermic effect of feeding, and directly, when I showed why getting 30 percent of your calories from protein works far better for weight control and body composition than does getting the standard amount of protein, which is about 15 percent of calories.

What I didn't mention is the utter weirdness of the arguments against eating more protein.

In the spring of 2006, I contributed some exercise and nutrition tips to a short article in *Esquire* magazine. I was amused to see my advice alongside that of a nutritionist declaring "the typical American already eats more protein than even elite athletes need."

That's only true if you define "need" as the minuscule quantity it takes to avoid turning our bodies into quivering blobs of gelatinous protoplasm. I concede that point, but I'd rather tell you how much protein produces the greatest benefit in terms of health and weight control. On that point, as I've noted, the research is consistent and unambiguous when it shows that women do best with about twice as much protein as the average American woman currently eats.

If you took the anti-protein argument to other areas of your life, and defined "need" as the bare minimum for survival, you'd quit your job (you don't need to work that hard to afford enough food to keep from starving), you'd move out of your house and into your storage shed (all you need is protection from the elements), you'd throw out all your possessions aside from one set of clothes (you can only wear one set at a time, so why have more?), and of course you'd only eat enough food to avoid starvation—which works out nicely, since that's all you can afford now.

Curiously, the people who speak of protein in terms of the minimum needed for survival don't extend their logic to the discussion of carbohydrates. (They used to talk about fat that way, but stopped when it became clear the obesity epidemic had nothing to do with that much-demonized macronutrient.) So what is it about protein that inspires this enmity?

It seems to start with the idea that public health would improve in a dramatic way if we ate less food from animals and more food from plants. But as I noted earlier in this chapter, there's really no long-term advantage to choosing one over the other. There is, however, a considerable *immediate* advantage to eating animal protein.

Protein is not an all-or-nothing macronutrient. There are twenty amino acids, the building blocks of protein, and you'll find them in different configurations in different foods. Animal proteins are complete, meaning they have all twenty aminos. Vegetable proteins tend to be incomplete, which is why you need rice with beans to get the full complement of amino acids in the same meal.

Not all amino acids are equal. Your body can make eleven of them even in the absence of dietary protein, just as it can run your brain on sugar without you eating any carbohydrates at all. That leaves nine that have to show up in your diet somewhere. Those are called "essential" amino acids—they're the protein equivalents of omega-6 and omega-3 polyunsaturated fats, which are likewise essential because your body can't make them from other fats.

Three of those nine fall into an even more exclusive category called "branched-chain amino acids." One of those, leucine, stands above the rest. Foods with the most leucine include the ones that are universally acknowledged as best for building muscle:

- cottage cheese and other dairy products
- eggs (most of the leucine is in the whites)

- turkey breast
- fish (especially tuna and cod)
- beef, chicken, pork, shellfish, and whatever other animal protein you might come across

Soy protein is the best vegetarian source of leucine, and is considered the best nonanimal protein source overall. However, if you use a standard called "biological value" to rate protein sources—that is, if you measure a food's protein quality as well as a human body's ability to use it—then soy finishes far below eggs, milk, fish, beef, and chicken. The food with the highest biological value ever measured is whey protein, which is used in many nutritional supplements (and recommended in Cassandra's diet plans in the next chapter).

No ranking method is perfect, nor is it vital to your health to know, say, that beef is ranked slightly higher than chicken in terms of biological value. The key is to understand that the results of your workouts can be enhanced or deflated by the quality of your diet in general, and the quality of protein in your diet in particular.

And that's a point that the protein minimalists consistently fail to tell whoever's listening to their advice. Your body is breaking down and building up muscle tissue all day, every day. This process accelerates when you work out with weights—you break down muscle tissue much faster, and also build it up much faster if you have enough protein when your body needs it most.

Furthermore, there's an additive effect of high-quality protein and strength training that's greater than the simple sum of strength-training benefits + high-quality-protein benefits. It's sort of like Fred Astaire and Ginger Rogers. Each is terrific individually, but the combination of the two is transcendent.

Cassandra's diet plans load up on the highest-quality protein sources—not much point in praising them if we aren't going to show you how to use them, right? But if you're unable to eat some of them—if you're lactose-intolerant and can't have dairy foods, for example—then soy protein is an acceptable substitute. Finally, if you're a vegetarian or vegan for religious or moral reasons, forget everything I just said and go for soy and any other vegetable proteins you can get your hands on. I have strong opinions, but they all come with the caveat "All things being equal." If you have reasons for not eating animal products, then all things aren't equal, and you have to develop an alternative nutrition strategy.

LIQUOR IS QUICKER

Alcohol is the odd duck of nutrition science. Technically, it's a carbohydrate, but its thermic effect is like that of protein, with up to 30 percent of its calories burned off in digestion. It has more calories per gram than carbohydrates—7 for alcohol, 4 for carbs—which makes it more like fat (9 calories per gram) than any other macronutrient.

Unlike protein, which in most studies appears to reduce appetite, alcohol may actually increase the amount of food you eat at any given meal. Even worse, your body will always process alcohol calories before any other type, since it can't store them. So your body will use less fat for energy when you have booze in your system.

You'd think that the people who drink the most would weigh the most, but studies haven't shown a connection between weight and calories from alcohol. One study showed that the most indulgent drinkers are more active than those who drink less, which the researchers offered as a possible explanation for why all that liquor wasn't making people thicker. The men and women in that study had, on average, one to two drinks per day, with alcohol accounting for 5 to 6 percent of their total daily calories. The researchers estimated that physical activity increased 3 percent for every 1 percent increase in the percentage of calories from alcohol in their diets.

I'd be tempted to write off the latter results as some kind of aberration, but I can recall seeing several major studies that showed similar trends. Once you get into the charts and graphs, you notice that those who burn the most calories in exercise also consume the most alcohol. I can't recall any other researchers flagging that as a major finding, but I've seen it more than once in the eyestrain-inducing small type.

I wish I could tell you what all this means for your physique. People in the body-transformation biz tend to advise their clients to minimize alcoholic intake, especially from beer and high-calorie mixed drinks. But I suspect you don't need a book to tell you that Kahlúa and cream won't help you get sleeker and stronger.

Red wine seems to be the best choice, with few calories, few carbohydrates, and some healthful micronutrients. Antioxidants called polyphenols, which originate in the grape skins that give the wine its color, are thought to help prevent cancer. I don't recommend drinking a lot of it, especially if a review of the data from your own history suggests that each glass of wine consumed at dinner makes you 20 percent more likely to have cheesecake for dessert.

Personally, I limit my consumption of wine to special occasions, although I grant myself a flexible definition of "special." Sometimes holidays aren't special enough, and sometimes I feel like celebrating just because it's Wednesday. My overall goal is to make sure one special evening doesn't extend into two or three special evenings in a row. Inevitably, I can feel it on my waistline.

Cassandra's meal plan allows for an occasional glass of wine, but if it's more than occasional, it may end up being more trouble than it's worth.

Our Meal Plans Can Beat Up Their Meal Plans

Before we offer suggestions on what to eat, we need to figure out how much to eat. I'll confess right up front that we're going to use rough estimates here. The numbers we use—and by "we," I mean Cassandra—are based on the Owen equation, one of several ways to estimate your resting metabolic rate without access to high-tech equipment.

The number you get by using the formula isn't pulled out of thin air—the Owen equation ranked as the best for normal-weight women in at least one study. But there is no single measure that works best for all women. Other formulas are considered better for obese women, for example, or for different ethnic groups, or for athletes.

And then there's the issue of the amount of activity you get in a day, and how much you move in general. Studies have shown that people who fidget burn more calories throughout the day than people who don't. Drinking water, chewing gum, sleeping more or less than usual . . . we could probably come up with dozens of reasons why you or anyone else would have a metabolic rate that's different from the ones the formulas predict.

Our goal is to give you a starting point, after which you can manipulate calories up or down, depending on how the initial calculation works out for you. We'll give you detailed instructions on how to cut calories if your calculations suggest you should (as I wrote earlier, I think we're all pretty proficient at adding them), and how often. First, though, let's establish some baseline numbers.

THE STARTING LINE

In the following example, I'm using a fictional woman who's five-foot-four, 140 pounds, and thirty years old.

Step 1. Weight in kilograms

Weigh yourself. First thing in the morning is best. Now divide that number by 2.2 to get your weight in kilograms. Our 140-pound woman weighs 63.64 kilograms, which I'm rounding up to 64.

Step 2. Resting metabolic rate

Run this equation:

$$795 + (7.18 \times \text{body weight in kilograms}) = \text{resting metabolic rate}$$

Our sample woman has a resting metabolic rate of 1,254 calories. That's the number of calories she'd burn if she did nothing and ate nothing all day. (If you're wondering where the constants in that equation—795 and 7.18—come from: The researchers start with an accurate measure of the resting metabolic rates of the subjects in their studies, using high-tech equipment with tongue-twisting names like "indirect calorimeter." Then they find the mathematical formula that most accurately predicts those metabolic rates.)

Step 3. Body mass index

Find your body mass index, or BMI, in the following table. BMI is a height-and-weight calculation that doesn't take into account your ratio of fat to muscle. So, like everything else in this chapter so far, it's more useful in general than it is when we're talking about a specific person.

Our five-foot-four sample, at 140 pounds, has a BMI of 24.

BMI	19	20	21	22	23	24	25	26	27	28	29	30	31	32	33	34	35
Height (feet-inches)								**Weight in pounds**									
4-10	91	96	100	105	110	115	119	124	129	134	138	143	148	153	158	162	167
4-11	94	99	104	109	114	119	124	128	133	138	143	148	153	158	163	168	173
5-0	97	102	107	112	118	123	128	133	138	143	148	153	158	163	168	174	179
5-1	100	106	111	116	122	127	132	137	143	148	153	158	164	169	174	180	185
5-2	104	109	115	120	126	131	136	142	147	153	158	164	169	175	180	186	191
5-3	107	113	118	124	130	135	141	146	152	158	163	169	175	180	186	191	197
5-4	110	116	122	128	134	140	145	151	157	163	169	174	180	186	192	197	204
5-5	114	120	126	132	138	144	150	156	162	168	174	180	186	192	198	204	210
5-6	118	124	130	136	142	148	155	161	167	173	179	186	192	198	204	210	216
5-7	121	127	134	140	146	153	159	166	172	178	185	191	198	204	211	217	223
5-8	125	131	138	144	151	158	164	171	177	184	190	197	203	210	216	223	230
5-9	128	135	142	149	155	162	169	176	182	189	196	203	209	216	223	230	236
5-10	132	139	146	153	160	167	174	181	188	195	202	209	216	222	229	236	243
5-11	136	143	150	157	165	172	179	186	193	200	208	215	222	229	236	243	250
6-0	140	147	154	162	169	177	184	191	199	206	213	221	228	235	242	250	258

Step 4. Daily-activities multipliers

Now, use your BMI and age to figure out how many calories you burn on two different days, depending on whether or not you work out. You'll notice the chart has an extra line labeled "strenuous work and workout day." If you're really active throughout the day—you work in construction, say, or you play a competitive sport with an hour or more of daily practice—and work out that same day, you'll multiply by a higher number than you would if you have a typical desk job.

	BMI 18 to 24.9		BMI > 25	
	Under 35 yrs	Over 35 yrs	Under 35 yrs	Over 35 yrs
No workout	1.6	1.4	1.5	1.2
Active workout day	1.8	1.6	1.7	1.4
Strenuous work and workout day	2.0	1.8	1.9	1.6

Since our sample woman is under thirty-five and has a BMI below 25, she'll multiply her resting metabolic rate—1,254—by 1.6 for nonworkout days and by 1.8 for the days she hits the weights. That gives her an expected calorie expenditure of 2,000 calories on the days she doesn't work out, and 2,257 when she does.

Step 5. Adjust for your goals

The two numbers we calculated probably look humongous to anyone who's ever read diet books, which typically prescribe meal plans of 1,200 to 1,400 calories a day for women. But these aren't *really* huge numbers. They're just what we expect our sample woman to burn on two typical days when she isn't trying to lose weight.

And if she is trying to lose weight?

Let's start with what we don't recommend. We don't want her to start off by slashing her daily calories by 500, which is the most common advice I've seen in my fifteen-plus years of writing about exercise and nutrition. (My coauthors and I even offered that advice in *Testosterone Advantage Plan*.) Why 500? Because a pound of fat contains 3,500 calories, which means that cutting 500 calories a day produces a pound a week of fat loss.

In theory, anyway.

The reality is that no one can predict the effects of a sudden decrease in energy intake. In our example, we're talking about a quarter of her daily calories. On the one hand, it's certainly going to be a shock to the system, and probably would produce some immediate weight loss. She might even be able to do the workouts in this book for a week or two.

After that, the prognosis isn't good.

Remember what I said in Chapter 4, about how the combination of "Eat less" and "Exercise more" is the physiological equivalent of "I voted for it before I voted against it"? Her body won't like the simultaneous stresses of less food—25 percent less—and more exercise. Even if the total amount of exercise she's doing on Alwyn's programs is less than she's used to, there's still going to be a real challenge to her body. The whole point of *New Rules* is to get her—in other words, you—to lift heavier weights, to do more challenging exercises, to develop total-body strength, and to add muscle mass—all of which will be severely compromised by a sudden drop in the amount of energy you give your body to work with.

Consider this:

It takes about 2,800 calories to build a pound of muscle. If you're slicing 3,500 calories a week from your diet while at the same time engaging in a workout program designed to increase strength and thus build new muscle tissue, from where will you get those 2,800 calories? My guess is that you'd actually lose muscle if you did these workouts with a 500-calorie-a-day deficit.

Let's look at it another way. You need 454 grams of protein to create a pound of muscle tissue. If you're eating 2,000 calories a day, and 30 percent of those come from protein, that's 4,200 calories a week from protein, or 1,050 grams. But if you cut down to 1,500 calories a day, and keep protein intake constant at 30 percent of total calories, you're now getting 3,150 calories a week from protein, or 787 grams.

That looks like enough to build muscle . . . until you consider that your body is already shedding and adding protein to your muscles every minute of every day. The technical phrase is "protein turnover." It happens even if you don't exercise—and if you do, the process accelerates. That's why 787 grams of protein isn't nearly enough to support exercise-induced protein turnover while giving you a net gain in muscle size.

I know I'm hitting you with a lot of numbers here, so let's see if we can simplify things by putting some rough estimates into chart form. I'm going to use three estimates of a strength-training athlete's protein needs: one minimal, one at the high end, and one in between. The low estimate comes from an older study, showing the rock-bottom needs of competitive bodybuilders who weren't cutting calories. The high estimate is commonly suggested for men and women who are trying to lose weight without losing muscle size. And, for the sake of simplicity, I chose a third number that's right down the middle of the two estimates. Once again, I'll use a 140-pound woman as an example.

Protein needs:
Low: 0.5 grams per pound of body weight per day, or 70 grams
Medium: 0.75 grams per pound of body weight per day, or 105 grams
High: 1 gram per pound of body weight per day, or 140 grams

Protein in 30% protein diet:
1,500 calories per day: 112 grams
2,000 calories per day: 150 grams

Estimated protein surplus/deficit, 1,500 calories/day:
Low-needs estimate: surplus of 52 grams of protein per day
Medium-needs estimate: surplus of 7 grams of protein per day
High-needs estimate: deficit of 28 grams of protein per day

Estimated protein surplus/deficit, 2,000 calories/day:
Low-needs estimate: surplus of 80 grams of protein per day
Medium-needs estimate: surplus of 45 grams of protein per day
High-needs estimate: surplus of 10 grams of protein per day

I hope your eyeballs aren't bleeding from all these numbers I'm throwing around. My point is simple: If our sample woman is eating 1,500 calories a day, the best she can hope for is that she breaks even—her body uses as much protein as she eats, and no more.

But that's unrealistic, for two reasons:

First, it's unlikely that her body would need just 70 grams of protein a day on a weight-loss diet. Remember, she's used to having 2,000 calories a day. That's her baseline, her point of homeostasis. Cut 500 calories, and suddenly her body is looking for energy wherever it can find it, and that probably means she'll use some of that dietary protein for energy.

Second, it's entirely possible that she'll use some of the protein *already stored in her muscles* to make up for the energy deficit. Everyone who's ever cut calories on a diet fantasizes that her body will use stored body fat to replace the missing energy, but the reality is that muscle is lost along with fat. The only way to preserve muscle tissue when drastically cutting calories is to eat a lot of protein. There's no way to know this for sure, but I'd guess that even the highest estimate of protein needs that I've shown here—140 grams of protein a day, which is 560 calories, or 37 percent of a 1,500-calorie-a-day diet—would be cutting it close.

And even then, it would be nearly impossible to add any muscle tissue.

Now let's assume she's eating 2,000 calories a day. On Cassandra's meal plans, she'd be getting about 150 grams of protein a day (with more on workout days, as I'll explain later in the chapter). That's gives her plenty of calories and protein to build muscle. Even if she works out like a madwoman on Alwyn's programs and burns off more energy than she takes in, she has her body's fat stores to fall back on. Thus, in theory, she could strip some fat and gain muscle without even cutting calories from her baseline needs.

Yes, "in theory" that could happen. But you want a bit more certainty, don't you? Let's discuss.

THE FIRST CUT

My initial instinct is to suggest that you don't try to cut calories at all at first. You'd calculate your maintenance level, and then stick with that for four weeks. That would take most of you through most of Phase 1 of the workout program, as well as keeping you at a single calorie level through an entire menstrual cycle.

I recommend that for three reasons:

1. We have no idea if that's your real maintenance level. It is, as I said, just a paper-and-pencil estimate.
2. You probably don't know if the predicted maintenance level is more than you're used to eating, less, or about the same.
3. You don't know how your body will react to Alwyn's workouts. Even if you're used to hard workouts, these are designed to produce metabolic perturbation— to shake things up. And if you aren't used to hard workouts, they'll *really* shake things up. That's not an optimal time to cut calories.

Ideally, after four weeks with maintenance-level calories, you'd assess your progress, based on these criteria:

- Did you gain weight, lose weight, or stay the same?
- Do your clothes feel loose, or are they tighter?
- Do you see any differences when you look in the mirror?
- How do you feel? Energized, or tired?
- How are your workouts going? Are you getting stronger from one workout to the next?
- How are you sleeping at night? Are you so tired you're falling asleep as soon as

your head hits the pillow? Do you feel anxious or jittery? Or has nothing changed?

- Has your menstrual cycle changed?

Let's look at what these signs indicate:

Weight

Weight gain is clearly a sign that you're eating more calories than you need to maintain your weight. If you were a guy like me, you'd be happy about that, since the combination of diet and exercise produced an increase in muscle mass. But I'd expect few of you to react that way, even if you suspected all the weight you'd gained was in the form of muscle mass. Weight loss is probably a good sign, unless you also feel chronically sluggish. (See below.) And weight maintenance could be good, bad, or neutral, depending on what else is going on.

Clothes

I don't need to tell you that loose-fitting jeans are a good sign, as are shirts that feel a bit more snug in the shoulders. If everything feels tighter but your scale weight hasn't changed, you're probably holding water, which is most likely temporary. If your scale weight hasn't changed but your clothes feel looser, you've hit the jackpot—you've lost fat and gained muscle, which takes up less space beneath your skin.

Visual differences

These are tricky. When our bodies change, they do so at such a slow pace that it's hard to tell just by looking in a mirror. Sometimes the best way to judge is to look in someone else's mirror. I'm more likely to notice changes in my physique—good or bad—when I see my reflection from an angle I can't see at home.

Friends and coworkers are also a good barometer of your progress. Compliments are rarely idle; if someone mentions a change in your appearance, it's because there's been a change in your appearance—the good kind. (I hope you don't have friends who'd mention a negative change, unless you brought it up first.)

Conversely, not hearing compliments isn't necessarily a sign that you're spinning your wheels. Husbands and boyfriends who see you every day won't notice the subtle changes that take place early in a new program. (They might not notice dramatic changes, either, but that's a different book.) And male coworkers could be afraid to mention positive changes in your appearance, for fear of crossing a line into the realm of unwanted attention. ("Barbara, your legs look sensational! And check out those glutes!")

Mood and energy level

You should never feel like you're running on fumes, in the gym or anywhere else. We all have our low-energy days, but if you're having more of them than usual, you have to at least consider the possibility that you're undernourished.

Strength

Here's an absolute: If you aren't getting progressively stronger during the first four weeks of Alwyn's workouts, something is wrong. Either you're not pushing yourself hard enough, or you used weights that were too heavy at the start of the program and did more harm than good, or you're not treating your body right outside the gym (drinking too much, working too hard, not sleeping enough . . .), or you aren't eating enough food to allow your body to recover between workouts.

Sleep

If you're so exhausted at the end of the day that you're almost asleep before you reach your bed, well, to tell you the truth, that sometimes happens when you're just starting a good training program. The key is that you actually sleep long and deeply once you go horizontal. If your pulse is racing at bedtime and you struggle to get into or stay in a deep sleep, you could be overtraining. That is, you aren't getting enough recovery between workouts, and you need to find a way to balance the stresses in your life. (Yes, I know how absurd it is for a man to say that to a woman. My wife has explained all this to me in vivid detail.)

It's also possible that not eating enough is keeping you awake at night.

I mentioned a racing pulse. One great way to gauge your reaction to the diet and workouts—and to tune into your body in general—is to monitor your resting pulse rate. Count the number of beats for 15 seconds, then multiply by four. It's best to do this first thing in the morning—before you even get out of bed, if possible—and also at night, just before you fall asleep. You don't have to do this daily. Just get a reading before you start the program, and then recheck it occasionally as you go along. You want it to go down (a sign of improved fitness) or stay the same. If it's rising, that's a sign of too much stress and too little recovery.

Menstrual cycle

This is more related to long-term undereating than anything that would happen in just four weeks. Still, it's something worth noting for future reference. If your cycles are normally predictable but suddenly get longer or become unpredictable, that could be a sign you're affecting your hormones by undereating.

Conversely, if your periods are typically erratic and unpredictable, but suddenly become more regular, you can probably assume that a better eating plan had a role.

Now, having advocated an ideal—start off with maintenance-level calories, and assess after four weeks—I'll get back to reality. I may not be the brightest bulb on the Christmas tree, but even I know that every woman in America—if not all of Western civilization—has been conditioned to think she must cut calories. So here's my suggestion for a calorie-management strategy:

- If you feel that you must eat below your predicted maintenance level, cut a maximum of 300 calories a day.
- No matter what, eat more calories on workout days than on nonworkout days. (I'll explain all that in the next section of this chapter.)
- Reassess your strategy after four weeks. Ask yourself the questions listed previously. If anything is affected negatively by your decision to cut calories—if you're chronically tired, having lousy or unproductive workouts, and losing sleep because of recurring nightmares involving malevolent pastries—then you need to increase your calories until the problems go away. That is, eat more *high-quality* calories from all three macronutrients; adding a bag of Doritos is unlikely to help you reach your goals.

INTRODUCING THE MEAL PLANS

The nutrition program Cassandra designed is completely modular. There are six meal categories:

- Breakfast
- Midmorning/midafternoon snacks
- Lunch
- Dinner

- Dessert
- Post-workout recovery shake

Within each category, you'll find a range of options listed by number of calories. Some are quick and easy to prepare, while others require more planning, prep work, and cooking time. You can put them together any way you want, based on your food preferences and the number of calories you choose as your daily target. You can also do simple multiplication to expand these meals so they feed friends and family, if that's an issue.

If you're a light breakfast eater, you can choose a lower-calorie morning meal, and then higher-calorie meals later in the day to make up for it. Or you can go the opposite direction, and load up at breakfast while eating lighter at lunch and dinner.

Here are the ironclad rules:

- You must eat breakfast.
- You must eat a total of five meals and snacks a day.
- You must have a post-workout recovery shake on the days you lift.
- You must have more calories on the days you work out than on the days you don't. (Conveniently, the post-workout shake takes care of the calories.)

We encourage you to try different combinations, but we also understand how difficult it is to find time to shop for and then cook a lot of new dishes. Plus, I'd be lying if I said I do things that way. I have the same things for breakfast, snacks, and post-workout shakes just about every day of my life. Dinner is something delicious my wife has prepared, and lunch is whatever's left over from the previous night's dinner. My wife keeps some Kashi or Lean Cuisine frozen dinners for me to have for lunch when the leftover-dinner option is inoperative, and when all else fails there's always eggs and whole-wheat toast.

In other words, I'm the last guy in the world to lecture anyone on the importance of preparing elaborate meals three times a day.

That said, you'll find some great recipes and meal plans on the following pages, and I hope you try them all eventually.

Each meal includes a breakdown, in grams, of its protein, carbohydrate, and fat. You'll also find listings for fiber and saturated fat. Our goal with these meals isn't to get you to restrict yourself to these choices and only these choices. We hope you experiment with these meals at first, to see how different combinations of foods can add up to the same daily totals, and then branch out and put together your own plans, with your own recipes and combinations.

Fresh Powder

We recommend a recovery shake that includes whey-protein powder after each workout. On top of that, Cassandra includes whey protein in several of the recipes in the following section. Her meal plans also offer the option of having a pre-workout drink in place of one of your midmorning or midafternoon snacks. And you can also use protein-rich nutrition bars in place of those snacks.

Given all that, you might begin to wonder if Cassandra, Alwyn, and I are on the payroll of a supplement company.

We aren't, but we do have friends who work in that industry. And even if we didn't, we'd be just as enthusiastic about supplemental protein. It's convenient, easy to use, relatively inexpensive, and, depending on the brand, tasty. (I mention taste because the protein supplements that were around in my youth were really nasty concoctions. I doubt if my dog—an animal that forms its world view by sniffing things we humans avoid—would eat them.)

Our focus here is on whey protein, one of the two main proteins found in milk. (The other is casein, which is slower to digest than whey.) As I mentioned in Chapter 6, whey has the highest biological value of any protein—that is, your body can make better use of it than any other collection of amino acids, whether they come from animal or vegetable sources.

You can buy whey one of two ways:

- By itself, as a flavored powder (vanilla, chocolate, strawberry), with no other macronutrients.
- As a meal-replacement product, or MRP. (Actually, I have no idea what the P stands for. Protein? Powder? Product? Pathology? Your guess is as good as mine.) MRPs may have a combination of whey and casein, or just whey; they also have some carbs and fat. Often they even have added fiber. The idea, as the first two words of the name imply, is to replace an entire meal.

You can find protein supplements in many outlets—grocery stores, Wal-Mart, drugstores, health food stores like GNC. Your gym probably sells them as well. I've never seen them in a clothing store, but that could change if they get any more popular.

I'll be honest about this: The taste and quality change dramatically from brand to brand. Quality isn't something that's immediately apparent, or that can be judged solely on taste. (In my experience, some well-regarded brands don't taste great, although I've yet to try a poorly regarded brand that tasted good.) This is where price matters. The more expensive brands—including EAS, Biotest, MET-Rx, and MuscleTech, among many others—tend to have the best reputations for quality, and sometimes they're the best-tasting as well. While I fully admit I'm biased, I put the flavor of Biotest products at the top of the list. (I sometimes write for Biotest's website, t-nation.com, as do Alwyn and Cassandra.)

The only way to discover the products that taste best, and that work best for you, is to start with research online. What you find will be all over the place, and rarely objective. But you should see some consensus develop, at least in terms of brands and product lines. After that, it's trial and error. Some health food stores allow you to sample products by purchasing single-serving packets. It's more expensive to do it that way, but it's cost effective in the long run, since you'll be less likely to buy a lot of something that ends up expiring on your shelf.

Here are some of the ways to use protein supplements.

Post-workout recovery shakes

No blender

1 scoop whey-protein powder, any flavor
¾ cup skim milk

- Shake by hand; you can find shaker cups in just about any store that sells protein supplements. Have with a banana to provide extra carbohydrates. (The only time you want extra carbs is post-exercise, when the nutrients will help your muscles recover.)

275 calories; 29 grams protein; 36 grams carbs (2.5 grams fiber); 2 grams fat (1 gram saturated)

WITHOUT THE BANANA: *165 calories; 28 grams protein; 10 grams carbs (0 grams fiber); 2 grams fat (1 gram saturated)*

Slim-Fast Plus

1 11-oz. can Slim-Fast Meal Options ready-to-drink shake (flavor of choice)
1 scoop whey-protein powder (same flavor)

- Mix together in a shaker cup, or stir together in a regular glass.

COMBO: *335 calories; 31 grams protein; 44 grams carbs (5 grams fiber); 4 grams fat (2 grams saturated)*

SLIM-FAST ALONE: *220 calories; 10 grams protein; 40 grams carbs (5 grams fiber); 4 grams fat (2 grams saturated)*

Blended shakes

Strawberry-pineapple-orange

1 scoop strawberry whey-protein powder
1 cup Dole 100% pineapple-orange juice
Ice

- Put all ingredients in a blender and process until smooth.

215 calories; 24 grams protein; 27 grams carbs (0 grams fiber); 1 gram fat (0.5 gram saturated)

Strawberry-banana

1 scoop vanilla whey-protein powder
6 medium strawberries, hulled
1 medium banana
Water
Ice

- Put all ingredients in a blender and process until smooth.

230 calories; 23 grams protein; 35 grams carbs (5 grams fiber); 0 grams fat

Pre-workout shakes

If you're going to exercise in the next hour or so, you can have a pre-workout shake instead of a midmorning or midafternoon snack. Two options:

EAS Myoplex Light ready-to-drink shake

190 calories; 25 grams protein; 20 grams carbs (5 grams fiber); 2.5 grams fat (1 gram saturated)

PROLAB Naturally Lean Complex (packet), mixed in water

195 calories; 20 grams protein; 20 grams carbs (4 grams fiber); 4 grams fat (1 gram saturated)

Nutrition bars

At best, these are made with the same high-quality proteins you find in MRPs. At worst, they're candy bars with added protein. (Snickers even makes a meal-replacement bar.) Also, keep in mind the difference between cereal bars (such as NutriGrain) and bars meant for people who lift weights. Some bars are deceptively marketed. Kashi's GoLean bars, for example, are meant to evoke the company's excellent breakfast cereal, with its whole grains, fiber, and protein. But a 280-calorie bar has 49 grams of carbs, including 33 grams of sugar. That's more than twice the sugar you'd get in a calorie-matched portion of the cereal.

Two we like:

Atkins Advantage

220 calories; 20 grams protein; 20 grams carbs (7 grams fiber); 9 grams fat (4 grams saturated)

Biotest Metabolic Drive

220 calories; 20 grams protein; 25 grams carbs (4 grams fiber); 6 grams fat (4 grams saturated)

You can also make your own meal-replacement bars:

Peanut butter snack bar

(for 5 bars)
4 scoops chocolate whey-protein powder
⅔ cup ground flaxseed
⅓ cup water
4 Tbsp. smooth, natural peanut butter
1 package Splenda or stevia (optional)

- Mix all ingredients together in a large bowl. At first the mixture will seem too thick to stir, but it will loosen up into a doughlike texture. If it doesn't, you can add a tablespoon or two of water.

- Divide the mixture into 5 balls and shape each into a bar. Seal them in plastic wrap and store in the refrigerator or freezer. Eat one at a time for a high-protein snack with lots of healthy omega-3 fat.

258 calories; 21 grams protein; 12 grams carbs (2 grams fiber); 14 grams fat (1 gram saturated)

BREAKFAST

Yogurt with ricotta cheese, fruit, and nuts

6 oz. (¾ cup) plain low-fat yogurt, or no-sugar-added low-fat yogurt
⅓ cup part-skim ricotta cheese
⅓ cup fresh (or frozen and thawed) blueberries
⅛ cup unsalted chopped walnuts (roughly 10 halves)

- Mix together in a bowl.

330 calories; 19 grams protein; 23 grams carbs (3 grams fiber); 18 grams fat (6 grams saturated)

High-fiber cereal with milk and extra protein

1 scoop vanilla whey-protein powder
¾ cup 1% milk
¾ cup Fiber One cereal
1 Tbsp. plumped seedless raisins

- Mix whey protein with milk, then pour over cereal and raisins.

300 calories; 33 grams protein; 33 grams carbs (21 grams fiber); 4 grams fat (2 grams saturated)

Hearty protein oatmeal

⅓ cup dry steel-cut oats (or old-fashioned oats)
½ cup 1% milk
1 scoop chocolate or vanilla whey-protein powder
1 Tbsp. sliced almonds

● Cook oats on a stove or in microwave with water, according to package directions. After cooking, add milk, protein powder, and almonds.

300 calories; 32 grams protein; 28 grams carbs (4 grams fiber); 7 grams fat (2 grams saturated)

Oatmeal protein pancakes

4 egg whites (or ½ cup liquid egg substitute)
¼ cup dry steel-cut oats (or old-fashioned oats)
2 Tbsp. vanilla whey-protein powder
2 Tbsp. whole-wheat pancake mix
½ banana, sliced
Dash cinnamon

● Put all ingredients in a bowl and mix. Spray skillet with cooking spray and cook mixture as you do regular pancakes. Serve with sugar-free syrup, or 1 tablespoon sugar-free applesauce.

355 calories; 39 grams protein; 43 grams carbs (5 grams fiber); 3 grams fat (1 gram saturated)

Iced protein coffee with whole-wheat bagel and light cream cheese

½ cup cold coffee
½ cup 1% milk
1 scoop vanilla whey-protein powder
Ice cubes
½ whole-wheat bagel, toasted
1 Tbsp. light, soft cream cheese

- Combine and stir the coffee, milk, and protein powder. Pour over ice cubes. Serve with half a bagel and light cream cheese.

350 calories; 35 grams protein; 44 grams carbs (3 grams fiber); 4 grams fat (3 grams saturated)

Breakfast shake

1 cup water
1 scoop chocolate or vanilla whey-protein powder
1 Tbsp. smooth natural peanut butter
½ cup dry steel-cut oats (or old-fashioned oats)

- Put all ingredients in a blender and process until smooth.

355 calories; 30 grams protein; 32 grams carbs (5 grams fiber); 12 grams fat (1 gram saturated)

White Lightning

At this late stage in the nutrition wars, I don't imagine you need Cassandra and me to tell you that some beverages have calories. With two or three clicks on the Starbucks website, you can learn that a Cinnamon Dolce Frappuccino Grande with whipped cream has 420 calories, including a whopping 53 grams of sugar.

Click around on the Snapple website, and you learn that a 16-ounce mint iced tea has 220 calories, with 25 grams of sugar. And a 12-ounce Mountain Dew has 165 calories, with 46 grams of sugar.

If you have a need for caffeine—a stimulant my coauthors and I hold in high esteem—you can get just about any beverage you want without the sugar, if you're willing to switch to diet drinks, or add artificial sweeteners to your coffee or tea. Again, we have no problems with that. If all the Internet rumors about how artificial sweeteners convert to formaldehyde in your body were true, I'd have embalmed myself ages ago.

There seems to be little downside, and plenty of benefit, to having some caffeine. And I have to think that if there were any serious health risks from artificial sweeteners, we'd know about them by now. Compared to the real health risks associated with real sweeteners (diabetes, obesity, heart disease), it's hard to get worked up about the alleged dangers of NutraSweet or Splenda. Another option is stevia, an herb extract that's three hundred times sweeter than sugar, but doesn't have any significant effect on blood chemistry. (It's sold as a nutritional supplement in the United States.)

Shell Stocked

Not only are eggs a great and inexpensive source of muscle-building protein, they're as versatile as anything you'll find in your local grocery store.

You'll note that the first of the four recipes below uses egg whites only, and the second uses a combination of whole eggs and egg whites. We don't mean to imply that the yolk is bad for you. It's actually rich in vitamins, and more than half the fat is monounsaturated. Most of that is oleic acid, the same healthy fat you find in olive oil. The rest of the fats are a combination of saturated and polyunsaturated.

Cassandra uses egg whites (or egg substitutes) in some recipes for taste and to manage the overall calories and fat content in the meals.

Here are four ways to egg yourself on.

Scrambled egg whites with toast and jam

6 egg whites, or ¾ cup Better'n Eggs (or another egg substitute)

2 mushrooms, sliced

⅓ cup chopped kale or spinach

2 Tbsp. minced fresh parsley

1 Tbsp. sunflower-seed kernels, roasted

½ cup mild salsa (look for one with no sugar added to the ingredients)

1 slice sprouted-grain bread (or 100% whole-grain bread), toasted

1 Tbsp. sugar-free, natural jam (such as Smucker's)

• Scramble the eggs with the veggies, parsley, and sunflower seeds. Top with the salsa. Serve with the toast and jam.

305 calories; 27 grams protein; 38 grams carbs (10 grams fiber); 5 grams fat (2 grams saturated)

Omelet topped with salsa

Olive oil or canola oil cooking spray

2 medium eggs

2 egg whites, or ⅓ cup Better'n Eggs (or another egg substitute)

⅓ cup chopped red tomatoes

1 Tbsp. chopped green onion

2 Tbsp. chopped fresh parsley
3 mushrooms, chopped
¼ cup shredded low-fat cheddar cheese
⅓ cup mild salsa (look for one with no sugar added to the ingredients)
½ cup canned pineapple (in juice, not syrup)

- Spray skillet with cooking spray and turn to medium-high heat. Mix together eggs and pour into skillet. While cooking, add tomatoes, green onion, parsley, mushrooms, and cheese.
- After cooking, slide omelet onto a plate, and top with salsa. Place the pineapple in a side dish.

300 calories; 26 grams protein; 22 grams carbs (2 grams fiber); 12 grams fat (4 grams saturated)

Breakfast Burrito

1 8-in. whole-wheat flour tortilla (soft taco size)
Olive oil or canola oil cooking spray
½ green onion, chopped
⅓ red ripe tomato, chopped
Salt and pepper, to taste
2 medium eggs, beaten
1 Tbsp. grated low-fat cheddar cheese
⅓ cup chopped fresh cilantro

- Place tortilla between two damp paper towels and microwave 20 seconds. This makes it softer and easier to roll.
- Spray a medium skillet with cooking spray and turn to medium heat. Add green onion, tomato, and salt and pepper (if desired). Sauté 2 minutes. Add beaten eggs to mixture and stir until eggs are fully set.

Put shredded cheese into middle of tortilla, put eggs and veggies over cheese, sprinkle with cilantro, roll up tortilla, and microwave 30 seconds.

297 calories; 17 grams protein; 28 grams carbs (1 gram fiber); 13 grams fat (4 grams saturated)

Fried eggs and Canadian bacon

2 oz. (4 small slices) Canadian pork bacon

2 large eggs

1 medium apple, cored and sliced

• In small or medium skillet, grill Canadian bacon and fry eggs, then serve with sliced apple.

298 calories; 24 grams protein; 19 grams carbs (4 grams fiber); 14 grams fat (4 grams saturated)

MORNING/MIDAFTERNOON SNACKS

Most of these can be prepped before work and easily transported in Tupperware.

Red pepper and hummus dip

• Slice 1 red bell pepper into strips. Dip in ½ cup hummus (made with olive or canola oil, such as Tribe classic hummus).

215 calories; 8 grams protein; 19 grams carbs (5 grams fiber); 12 grams fat (1 gram saturated)

Fresh mozzarella and tomato with red wine vinaigrette dressing

⅓ cup extra-virgin olive oil

2 Tbsp. red wine vinegar

1 large clove garlic, crushed

⅓ cup minced fresh basil, or 1 Tbsp. dried

Salt and pepper, to taste

2 oz. (½ cup) part-skim mozzarella cheese, cut into small chunks

½ cup cherry tomatoes, cut in half

- In a small covered jar, combine oil, vinegar, garlic, basil, salt and pepper. Shake well to blend.
- Place mozzarella and tomatoes in a plate or bowl. Top with 1–2 tablespoons of the vinaigrette dressing. Chill 30 minutes before serving.

TOTAL MEAL: *205 calories; 16 grams protein; 6 grams carbs (1 gram fiber); 13 grams fat (8 grams saturated)*

Cottage cheese and raisins

1 cup 1% cottage cheese
1 Tbsp. plumped seedless raisins

- Mix ingredients together.

195 calories; 28 grams protein; 14 grams carbs (1 gram fiber); 3 grams fat (2 grams saturated)

Roast Likely to Succeed

Labels on packages of nuts can be hard to decipher. In our recipes, we use the word "natural" to mean raw, or "not roasted." If the package describes the nuts as "roasted," it means they've been cooked in vegetable oil. That changes the fat content, adding more omega-6 fatty acids than the nuts would have in their raw or natural state.

Roasted nuts aren't always labeled as such. Cashews, for example, might be sold as "unsalted," but if you look at the ingredients, you'll see "peanut and/or canola and/or cottonseed oil."

"Dry roasted" nuts, on the other hand, have no added oils.

Peanut butter labeled "natural" used to mean it contained nuts and perhaps a little salt, but nothing else. Now it can mean almost anything. One product calling itself "natural" has added sugar and palm oil. So read the label carefully before putting the nuts in your shopping cart.

Nuts and raisins

1 Tbsp. plumped seedless raisins
⅛ cup natural almonds (about 16 pieces)
⅛ cup unsalted pecan halves (about 11 pieces)

- Mix together or eat separately.

230 calories; 5 grams protein; 12 grams carbs (4 grams fiber); 18 grams fat (1 gram saturated)

Cottage cheese and cashews

½ cup 1% cottage cheese
¼ cup unsalted cashews (about 22 pieces)

- Mix together or eat separately.

220 calories; 18 grams protein; 8 grams carbs (1 gram fiber); 13 grams fat (3 grams saturated)

Chicken with crackers

8 Triscuit whole-wheat crackers
2 oz. (5 slices) low-fat chicken breast slices

215 calories; 12 grams protein; 26 grams carbs (4 grams fiber); 7 grams fat (1 gram saturated)

Midday shake

¾ cup 1% milk
1 scoop strawberry or vanilla whey-protein powder
2 Tbsp. fat-free plain yogurt
1 tsp. ground flaxseed (can buy already ground in select stores)
5 medium strawberries, hulled
Ice

- Whip all ingredients in a blender. Add water, if desired.

233 calories; 26 grams protein; 21 grams carbs (3 grams fiber); 5 grams fat (2 grams saturated)

Apple dipped in peanut butter

1 medium apple, sliced
2 Tbsp. smooth natural peanut butter

285 calories, 8 grams protein; 28 grams carbs (7 grams fiber); 16 grams fat (2 grams saturated)

Multigrain rice cakes topped with Swiss cheese and ham

3 oz. (about 4 slices) fat-free deli ham slices
2 oz. light Swiss cheese slices
2 large multigrain rice cakes
Dill weed, fresh or dried
Yellow mustard

● Place half the ham and Swiss cheese on each rice cake. Top with dill and mustard (or other seasoning/condiment of choice).

275 calories; 31 grams protein; 25 grams carbs (1 gram fiber); 6 grams fat (1 gram saturated)

High-protein yogurt with walnuts

½ cup fat-free plain yogurt
1 scoop vanilla whey-protein powder
⅛ cup natural unsalted chopped walnuts (roughly 10 halves)

● Mix the above together.

253 calories; 30 grams protein; 13 grams carb (1 gram fiber); 9 grams fat (1 gram saturated)

LUNCH

Greek salad with chicken

1½ cups red leaf lettuce, chopped
5 large pitted black olives, sliced

1 Tbsp. crumbled feta cheese

8 cherry tomatoes

3 oz. boneless, skinless chicken breast (roughly 1 medium-size breast), broiled or grilled

1 tsp. extra-virgin olive oil

2 Tbsp. balsamic vinegar

285 calories; 30 grams protein; 12 grams carbs (3 grams fiber); 13 grams fat (3 grams saturated)

Chef's salad

3 cups chopped romaine lettuce

1 medium hard-boiled egg

2 oz. (¾ of a breast) chicken, roasted, boneless, skinless

1 oz. (2 slices) low-fat cheddar cheese

1 oz. (2 slices) low-sodium ham

5 cherry tomatoes

½ small cucumber, peeled and sliced

1 Tbsp. light salad dressing made with olive oil (e.g., the red wine vinaigrette on pages 82–83)

310 calories; 35 grams protein; 11 grams carbs (4 grams fiber); 14 grams fat (4 grams saturated)

Tuna sandwich with small salad

¾ 6-oz. can chunk light tuna in water, drained (lowest in mercury)

1 tsp. light real mayonnaise

1 Tbsp. yellow mustard

1 tsp. chopped white onion

2 slices 100% whole-wheat bread

- Mix tuna with mayonnaise, mustard, and onion, then make a sandwich.

FOR SALAD, MIX TOGETHER:

1½ cups salad greens

3 mushrooms, sliced

½ Roma tomato, sliced

⅓ small cucumber, peeled and sliced

2 Tbsp. light salad dressing made with olive oil

320 calories; 31 grams protein; 31 grams carbs (5 grams fiber); 8 grams fat (1 gram saturated)

Tuna-apple-walnut salad

1 6-oz. can chunk light tuna in water, drained

5 cherry tomatoes

3 mushrooms, sliced

½ medium apple, cored, peeled, and sliced

⅛ cup (roughly 10 pieces) walnut halves

2 cups romaine lettuce leaves, chopped

2 Tbsp. Nakano light seasoned rice vinegar

- Put the tuna, veggies, apple, and nuts on top of the lettuce, then add the vinegar and toss.

320 calories; 34 grams protein; 23 grams carbs (5 grams fiber); 11 grams fat (1 gram saturated)

Quick vegetable soup with chicken and salmon

½ can Healthy Choice Garden Vegetable soup

3 oz. grilled chicken, chopped

3 oz. smoked salmon, chopped

- *On the stove:* Heat the soup on a stove in a small saucepan with the chopped chicken and salmon. Once heated, transfer to a soup bowl and enjoy.
- *In the microwave:* Place the soup into a microwavable container, and heat in the microwave according to the directions on the can. Heat the chicken and salmon until they're warm, and then mix them into the soup.

345 calories; 46 grams protein; 25 grams carbs (3 grams fiber); 7 grams fat (3 grams saturated)

Avocado-tuna salad

½ Hass avocado (3 oz.), peeled and cubed
½ small cucumber, peeled and diced
½ fresh red tomato, diced
½ cup canned black beans, rinsed and drained
½ 6-oz. can chunk light tuna in water, drained
1 Tbsp. balsamic vinegar (or to taste)
1 Tbsp. minced fresh oregano or 1 tsp. dried
1 Tbsp. minced fresh basil or 1 tsp. dried

● Mix ingredients together in a bowl.

● For a meal using the rest of the avocado, see the grilled turkey patty in the Dinner section.

372 calories; 25 grams protein; 32 grams carbs (14 grams fiber); 16 grams fat (2 grams saturated)

Need for Speed

Fast food isn't necessarily synonymous with junk food. True, most cuisine available at a drive-through window leaves a lot to be desired, nutritionally. And even the healthier choices tend to be a bit heavy on the sodium and highly processed carbohydrates, and light on whole grains and vegetables. But, you know, there are times when you have to settle for the least worst, instead of holding out for the best. We understand. We've been there. Here are six respectable choices from fast-food emporia.

Subway Turkey Breast Wrap

222 calories; 24 grams protein; 18 grams carbs (9 grams fiber); 6 grams fat (1 gram saturated)

Subway Oven Roasted Chicken Breast Sub (6 inches; no cheese)

330 calories; 24 grams protein; 47 grams carbs (4 grams fiber); 5 grams fat (1.5 grams saturated)

Quiznos Turkey Lite Sub (6 inches, wheat bread)

334 calories; 17 grams protein; 52 grams carbs (3 grams fiber); 6 grams fat (1 gram saturated)

Wendy's Roasted Turkey & Basil Pesto Frescata Sandwich

*420 calories; 21 grams protein; 50 grams carbs (4 grams fiber); 15 grams fat
(1 gram saturated)*

Wendy's Mandarin Chicken Salad (with berry balsamic vinegar dressing; without crispy noodles)

*390 calories; 27 grams protein; 34 grams carbs (6 grams fiber); 16 grams fat
(2 grams saturated)*

McDonald's Asian Salad with Grilled Chicken

*300 calories; 32 grams protein; 23 grams carbs (5 grams fiber); 10 grams fat
(1 gram saturated)*

Frozen Assets

Looking for something even faster? Frozen dinners work great with our meal-planning system; the nutrition info is on the box, so you can plug them right in. Our favorite frozen-meal lines are Kashi and Lean Cuisine. Two good choices:

Kashi Lime Cilantro Shrimp

*252 calories; 12 grams protein; 33 grams carbs (6 grams fiber); 8 grams fat
(2 grams saturated)*

Lean Cuisine Dinnertime Selects Balsamic Glazed Chicken

*380 calories; 18 grams protein; 60 grams carbs (4 grams fiber); 7 grams fat
(2.5 grams saturated)*

DINNER

Some of the following dinners are light (300 to 500 calories) and perfect for having as leftovers at lunch the next day. Others are more sumptuous (500+ calories) and include side dishes—salads, vegetables, starches (good to have an hour or two after lifting, when your body is still pushing nutrients to your muscles to help recover from the workout), and even wine in some cases.

For the bigger dinners, we include two nutrient breakdowns—one for the entire dinner, including the side dishes; and one for the main dish only, for when you have the leftovers at subsequent meals.

LIGHT DINNERS

Grilled shrimp with whole-wheat couscous

Serves 4

12 ounces large peeled shrimp

2 Tbsp. extra-virgin olive oil

4 Tbsp. lemon juice

2 Tbsp. chopped fresh parsley

2 Tbsp. minced fresh basil, or 2 tsp. dried

2 tsp. dried mustard

4 cloves garlic, minced

Pinch salt

¾ cup whole-wheat couscous (cooked) per serving

- Marinate shrimp for 1 to 2 hours in a mixture of the other ingredients. Grill shrimp 10 to 12 minutes, until thoroughly cooked.
- Place cooked shrimp over cooked couscous.

350 calories; 23 grams protein; 37 grams carbs (6 grams fiber); 13 grams fat (1 gram saturated)

Ground turkey chili

Serves 4

2 Tbsp. extra-virgin olive oil

½ cup diced yellow onion

4 cloves garlic, minced

½ lb. extra-lean ground turkey

1 6-oz. can tomato paste (no sugar added)

1 Tbsp. chili powder

2 tsp. ground cumin

1 15.5-oz. can dark kidney beans, rinsed and drained

1 14-oz. can diced tomatoes (no sugar added)

8 oz. sliced mushrooms

½ cup water

- In a medium nonstick saucepan, heat oil on medium-high. Add onion and garlic and sauté until golden. Add ground turkey and cook, breaking up the meat into crumbles with a wooden spoon, until meat is no longer pink.

- Add tomato paste, chili powder, and cumin. Sauté 1 minute. Add beans, tomatoes, mushrooms, and water. Simmer 10 to 15 minutes, until liquid is slightly reduced.

312 calories; 20 grams protein; 31 grams carbs (11 grams fiber); 12 grams fat (2 grams saturated)

Cooked lentils over mixed-green salad

Serves 4

1¼ cups dried green lentils (about 9 oz.), picked over to remove any stones

3 cloves garlic, peeled and crushed lightly

3 bay leaves

1 tsp. salt

3 medium carrots, peeled and diced fine (about 1 cup)

2 Tbsp. lemon juice

2 Tbsp. extra-virgin olive oil

1 medium celery stalk, diced fine (about ⅓ cup)

3 medium radishes, diced fine (about ⅓ cup)

2 Tbsp. minced fresh dill

Ground black pepper

8 cups mixed spring greens

4 oz. (about ¾ cup) crumbled feta cheese (full fat)

- Bring lentils, garlic, bay leaves, and 2 quarts water to a boil in medium saucepan over high heat. Reduce heat and simmer briskly 15 minutes.
- Stir in salt and carrots, and continue cooking about 10 minutes, until lentils and carrots are tender but not mushy. Drain and discard garlic and bay leaves.
- While lentils are cooking, remove 2 tablespoons cooking water from pot and transfer to medium bowl. Whisk in lemon juice, olive oil, and salt to taste.
- Add drained lentils, celery, radishes, and dill to bowl with lemon juice dressing. Toss to combine and then adjust seasonings, adding salt and pepper to taste. Let cool 5 minutes.
- Divide lentil mixture into 4 portions. Place each portion over 2 cups of mixed spring greens. Sprinkle 1 ounce of feta cheese over lentils.

317 calories; 20 grams protein; 30 grams carbs (12 grams fiber); 13 grams fat (5 grams saturated)

Slow-cooker spicy shrimp and chicken jambalaya; brown rice

Serves 6

1 lb. boneless, skinless chicken breast, cut into 1-inch cubes

2 14-oz. cans diced tomatoes with juice (no sugar added)

1 large onion, chopped

1 large green bell pepper, chopped

3 medium stalks celery, chopped

8 oz. sliced mushrooms

1 cup water

3 Tbsp. minced fresh oregano, or 2 tsp. dried

2 Tbsp. minced fresh parsley

2 tsp. Cajun seasoning

2 tsp. cayenne

1 Tbsp. minced fresh thyme, or ½ tsp. dried

2 bay leaves

1 lb. frozen, cooked, deveined shrimp without tails

½ cup brown rice (cooked) per serving

- Cook chicken to 80 percent doneness. Fill the slow cooker with everything *except* the shrimp and chicken, and set to low/medium heat and cook 3 hours.

- Add chicken and cook another 30 minutes. Add frozen shrimp and cook another 30 minutes.

- Remove bay leaves before serving. Serve ⅙ of jambalaya with ½ cup cooked brown rice.

385 calories; 46 grams protein; 39 grams carbs (7 grams fiber); 5 grams fat (1 gram saturated)

FULL DINNERS

Oregano chicken with fresh tomato-olive sauce, sweet potato french fries, and spinach salad with homemade vinaigrette

Serves 4

OREGANO CHICKEN WITH FRESH TOMATO-OLIVE SAUCE

1 cup cherry tomatoes, quartered

12 pitted black olives, coarsely chopped

2 Tbsp. coarsely chopped fresh parsley

1 Tbsp. cider vinegar

1 tsp. extra-virgin olive oil

1 clove garlic, diced

¼ tsp. salt

Olive oil or canola oil cooking spray

1 lb. chicken breast tenders

1 Tbsp. minced fresh oregano, or ½ tsp. dried

½ tsp. lemon-pepper seasoning

- In medium bowl, stir together tomatoes, olives, parsley, vinegar, oil, garlic, and salt; set aside. Warm a 12-inch nonstick skillet over medium heat. Remove from heat and spray with cooking spray. Add chicken to skillet. Sprinkle with oregano and lemon-pepper seasoning. Cook 5 minutes, or until no longer pink in center, turning frequently. Put ¼ of the chicken onto each plate and spoon ¼ of the tomato mixture over.

SWEET POTATO FRENCH FRIES

● Preheat oven to 475 degrees. Peel one medium sweet potato and slice lengthwise into ½-inch-wide strips. Place fries on nonstick baking sheet and spray fries with olive oil cooking spray. Lightly season with salt or other spices, as desired.

● Bake 20 to 30 minutes, or until crisped as desired. Serve fries with sugar-free or low-carb ketchup (such as Heinz One Carb Ketchup).

SPINACH SALAD AND HOMEMADE VINAIGRETTE

⅓ cup white vinegar
⅓ cup cider vinegar
1 Tbsp. paprika
1 Tbsp. extra-virgin olive oil
2 medium cloves garlic, finely chopped
¼ cup dry-roasted sunflower seed kernels
1 10-oz. bag baby spinach leaves
1 cup chopped cucumber
8 mushrooms, sliced

● In a small bowl, combine the first six ingredients.

● Pour mixture over spinach leaves mixed with cucumber and mushrooms. Toss.

FULL DINNER: *500 calories; 33 grams protein; 47 grams carbs (7.5 grams fiber); 21 grams fat (3 grams saturated)*

CHICKEN AND SPINACH SALAD ONLY (NO FRIES): *350 calories; 31 grams protein; 19 grams carbs (4 grams fiber); 17 grams fat (2 grams saturated)*

Orange-spiced salmon with peas and mixed-green salad

Serves 2
Olive oil or canola oil cooking spray
¼ cup unsweetened orange juice
2 Tbsp. lemon juice
2 6-oz. fresh salmon fillets with skin
½ tsp. paprika
½ tsp. curry powder
½ tsp. salt

¼ tsp. ground cinnamon

⅛ tsp. cayenne

Lemon juice, for sprinkling

- Preheat oven to 425 degrees. Line a baking sheet with aluminum foil. Lightly spray foil with cooking spray.
- In large resealable plastic bag, combine orange juice and lemon juice. Rinse salmon and add to juice mixture, turning several times to coat evenly. Seal bag and refrigerate 30 minutes, turning occasionally. (The timing is important; if you leave it in the marinade too long, the salmon will lose its firm texture.)
- In small bowl, mix together paprika, curry powder, salt, cinnamon, and cayenne; set aside.
- Remove salmon from bag and discard marinade. Arrange salmon skin-side down on prepared baking sheet. Rub or sprinkle dry spice mixture over salmon.
- Bake 14 minutes, or until salmon flakes easily when tested with a fork. To serve, place salmon on plates and sprinkle with lemon juice. Eat the skin for its rich source of omega-3 fatty acids.

PEAS AND MIXED-GREEN SALAD

1 cup frozen peas, steamed and drained

2 cups mixed salad greens

1 Tbsp. light salad dressing made with olive oil

FULL DINNER: *405 calories; 40 grams protein; 30 grams carbs (11 grams fiber); 14 grams fat (2 grams saturated)*

SALMON ONLY: *255 calories; 31 grams protein; 2 grams carbs (0 grams fiber); 11 grams fat (1.5 grams saturated)*

Pork chops with applesauce, steamed spinach, and three-bean salad

You'll need to prepare the three-bean salad several hours in advance, which makes this a good choice for weekends.

4 4-oz. lean, boneless pork chops

4 tsp. apple cider vinegar

Salt, to taste

4 Tbsp. unsweetened applesauce

● Broil pork chops, adding vinegar and salt to taste. Serve with applesauce on top of pork chops and a side of steamed spinach.

STEAMED SPINACH

● Take one 10-ounce bag fresh spinach and steam in 1 cup water in large pot on stove until leaves are wilted. Top with cider vinegar and salt to taste. (For a single serving, use one-quarter of the bag.)

THREE-BEAN SALAD

¼ cup red wine vinegar
3 Tbsp. extra-virgin olive oil
¾ tsp. Italian seasoning
1 small clove garlic, minced
¼ tsp. salt
⅛ tsp. black pepper
1 cup fresh green beans, steamed and cooled, or 1 cup frozen green beans, thawed
1 15-oz. garbanzo beans, rinsed and drained
1 15-oz. dark red kidney beans, rinsed and drained
¼ cup sliced green onions

● In large bowl, combine vinegar, olive oil, and seasonings; mix well. Stir in remaining ingredients. Refrigerate, covered, several hours or overnight, stirring occasionally.

FULL DINNER: *590 calories; 53 grams protein; 45 grams carbs (15 grams fiber); 22 grams fat (4 grams saturated)*

PORK CHOP AND APPLESAUCE ONLY: *215 calories; 36 grams protein; 2 grams carbs (0 grams fiber); 7.5 grams fat (2 grams saturated)*

THREE-BEAN SALAD ONLY: *236 calories; 13 grams protein; 37 grams carbs (12 grams fiber); 4 grams fat (1 gram saturated)*

Grilled turkey patty with tomato and avocado slices; black beans; mixed-green salad with balsamic dressing

4 oz. lean ground turkey
2 slices red tomato

1 slice (1 oz.) Hass avocado

Ketchup or mustard, to taste

½ cup (⅓ can) black beans, rinsed and drained

2 cups mixed salad greens

⅓ cup chopped red tomato

⅓ cup sliced, peeled cucumber

2 mushrooms, sliced

2 Tbsp. balsamic vinegar

- Form ground turkey into a patty. Cook on a grill until meat is no longer pink.
- Top patty with sliced tomato, avocado, and condiments. Serve with heated beans and the mixed salad on the side.

479 calories; 35 grams protein; 42 grams carbs (14 grams fiber); 19 grams fat (4 grams saturated)

Stir-fried steak; brown rice; red wine

Serves 4

¾ cup brown rice, uncooked

1 lb. top round steak

4 cups frozen Oriental stir-fry vegetables

8 Tbsp. Kikkoman less-sodium teriyaki marinade & sauce

- Cook brown rice according to package directions.
- Broil the steak to desired doneness, then cut into strips.
- Preheat skillet over medium-high heat. Add vegetables and a few tablespoons water. Don't overcook—you want them to stay crunchy. Reduce heat, add steak and teriyaki sauce, and heat until warm.
- Serve stir-fry over cooked rice. Enjoy with 4 ounces (½ cup) of your favorite red wine.

FULL DINNER: *525 calories; 42 grams protein; 43 grams carbs (3 grams fiber); 12 grams fat (3 grams saturated); 11 grams alcohol*

STEAK AND STIR-FRY VEGETABLES ONLY: *340 calories; 40 grams protein; 20 grams carbs (2 grams fiber); 11 grams fat (3 grams saturated)*

Glass Hassles

I recently traveled to St. Louis to help my siblings clear out and prepare our family home for sale. Our mother had lived in the five-bedroom house thirty-five years, and had recently downsized into a one-bedroom apartment.

As you can imagine, she left behind a lot of stuff she no longer needed, including a shelf full of wine and cocktail glasses of every shape and description. The first thing I noticed about the glasses is how small they were.

In her generation, a standard wineglass, used for white wine, held about 6 ounces—three-quarters of a cup. A four-ounce serving, recommended in several of these dinners, would occupy two-thirds of that glass, which is just about right. (You want to leave some room at the top to enjoy the bouquet.)

A bottle of wine is 750 milliliters, or 25.4 ounces. That means you'll get five to six four-ounce glasses per bottle.

Today, though, glasses are bigger—sometimes much bigger. A generation ago, a large red-wine glass held about nine ounces. If you filled it halfway, leaving plenty of room to swirl the wine to bring out the sensual nuances, you'd get four to five ounces per serving—about the same as you'd put in a smaller white-wine glass.

A red-wine glass today is more like a brandy snifter, holding fourteen ounces. So if you went by sight and filled that glass halfway, you'd be getting almost twice the serving size we recommend.

You may decide that you want more wine anyway. (I'll confess I'd have a hard time stopping at just four ounces.) The precise measurement at any given meal isn't as important as the practice of knowing how much of anything you're putting into your body.

Believe me, I know how geeky it is to measure wine before you pour it into a glass. But you only need to do it once, to see how four ounces or eight ounces or any other amount looks in your favorite wineglass. Even if it ends up looking like a puddle in the bottom of a fishbowl, at least you know how big the puddle is.

Poached halibut with herb-mustard sauce; brown rice; green beans; white wine

In France, fish is often cooked in barely simmering liquid. If you bring the liquid to a boil and then turn off the stove before adding the fish, the residual heat will cook the fish sufficiently. This technique keeps the fish from breaking apart as it cooks. Buying fish with the skin on also helps ensure that the fish remains intact.

The following recipe calls for simmering the fish in a mixture of water and white wine, but you can use a cup of water instead of the cup of wine, if you prefer.

Serves 4

1 cup white wine

2 tsp. salt

⅓ cup minced fresh parsley, or 1 Tbsp. dried

4 boneless, skin-on halibut steaks (5 oz. each raw)

⅓ cup minced fresh tarragon, or 1 Tbsp. dried

1 Tbsp. Dijon mustard

1 Tbsp. white wine vinegar

2 Tbsp. extra-virgin olive oil

Salt and ground black pepper, to taste

¾ cup brown rice (cooked) per serving

1 cup fresh green beans, steamed, or 1 cup frozen beans, steamed, per serving

- Bring wine, 4 cups water, 2 teaspoons salt, and parsley to a boil in large sauté pan. Remove pan from heat, slide fish into pan, cover, and set aside about 12 minutes, until fish is opaque throughout. (To judge doneness, slide a paring knife into the center and peek in.)

- Meanwhile, in medium bowl, mix tarragon, mustard, vinegar, and oil. Season with salt and pepper to taste.

- With slotted spatula, carefully lift halibut from poaching liquid, allowing liquid to drain back into pan. Place one piece of fish on each plate. Top each piece of fish with generous dollop of herb sauce. Serve immediately.

- Serve the halibut with sauce over the brown rice, with the green beans on the side. Enjoy with 4 ounces (½ cup) of white wine.

FULL DINNER: *535 calories; 39 grams protein; 44 grams carbs (7 grams fiber); 14 grams fat (2 grams saturated); 11 grams alcohol*

HALIBUT AND GREEN BEANS ONLY: *284 calories; 36 grams protein; 8 grams carbs (4 grams fiber); 12 grams fat (2 grams saturated)*

Spaghetti squash with ground-turkey tomato sauce

Serves 2

1 large spaghetti squash

2 tsp. extra-virgin olive oil

½ white onion, chopped

½ lb. lean ground turkey

2 cloves garlic, minced

1 14-oz. can diced tomatoes
1 zucchini, diced
⅓ cup minced fresh oregano, or 1 Tbsp. dried
2 Tbsp. fresh parsley
Salt and pepper, to taste
Parmesan cheese, freshly grated or dried

SPAGHETTI SQUASH:

* *To cook in the microwave:* Cut squash in half, lengthwise. Scoop out seeds. Microwave on High 12 to 16 minutes, with the cut side up. No need to cover. Using a fork, separate squash into strands, placing strands into a large bowl.
* *To cook in a conventional oven:* Preheat oven to 375 degrees. Clean the outside of the shell and then pierce several times with a large fork or skewer. Place in a baking dish and cook approximately 50 minutes, or until flesh is tender. Once cooked, let stand about 10 minutes until flesh has cooled, then cut in half and remove seeds. Using a fork, separate squash into strands, placing strands into large bowl.

TOMATO SAUCE

* Heat oil in saucepan. Add onion and stir until softened. Add ground turkey and cook, breaking up the meat into crumbles with a wooden spoon, until meat is no longer pink. Add garlic and cook 2 more minutes. Add tomatoes—including the juices in the can; in other words, don't drain.
* Bring to a simmer and stir in the zucchini, then the herbs. Simmer, uncovered, about 10 minutes, until sauce has thickened. Add salt and pepper to taste.
* Divide squash and sauce into equal portions. Place a portion of the squash on your plate, then top with a portion of the sauce. Sprinkle with Parmesan cheese.

500 calories; 32 grams protein; 50 grams carbs (6 grams fiber); 19 grams fat (5 grams saturated)

Herb-crusted salmon with asparagus; red wine

Serves 2
2 6-oz. salmon fillets with skin
1 tsp. salt
1 tsp. freshly ground pepper
2 tsp. Dijon mustard

1½ cups fresh assorted herbs such as parsley, basil, chervil, chives, tarragon, dill, or
    any other herb of your choice, chopped (or 2 Tbsp. dried mixed herbs)
1 Tbsp. butter
30 asparagus stalks, cleaned and ends snapped off
1 tsp. butter
Lemon wedges

- Preheat oven to 350 degrees.
- Sprinkle salmon on both sides with salt and pepper. Spread mustard on both
sides of each fillet, then dredge in chopped herbs and press herbs onto fillets with
your hands.
- Heat 1 tablespoon butter in a 10-inch, ovenproof, nonstick skillet over high heat
until very hot. Place salmon in skillet and cook about 1 minute per side, turning
carefully to preserve herb crust. Place skillet in preheated oven and roast about 5
minutes for medium, 10 minutes or longer for well done.
- While salmon is baking, steam asparagus. Then portion out 15 spears asparagus
per person and top with 1 teaspoon butter.
- Squeeze one fresh lemon wedge over each salmon fillet once it is cooked. Enjoy
with 4 ounces (½ cup) of red wine.

*560 calories; 50 grams protein; 14 grams carbs (5 grams fiber); 26 grams fat (9 grams
saturated); 10 grams alcohol*

Beer mussels with sweet potato and white wine

Serves 2
1 lb. raw mussels in shells
1 12-oz. can lager beer
Garlic powder
1 medium sweet potato

- Preheat oven to 350 degrees.
- Place mussels on large baking sheet. Pour beer over mussels, then sprinkle mussels with garlic powder. Cook 20 minutes. Remove from oven and let cool.
- *To cook sweet potato in microwave:* Cook sweet potato in the microwave, according
to manufacturer's directions.
- *To cook sweet potato in conventional oven:* Preheat oven to 375 degrees. Wash
potato lightly to remove dirt without breaking skin, then dry with a paper towel.

Pierce skin a couple of times with a fork to allow steam to escape. Place potato on a baking sheet and bake 45 to 55 minutes (depending on size of potato). Test potato for doneness by squeezing gently; when done, the potato will be slightly soft. Serve half the mussels with the potato, and enjoy with a 4-ounce glass of white wine.

560 calories; 56 grams protein; 45 grams carbs (4 grams fiber); 9 grams fat (2 grams saturated); 11 grams alcohol

Chili scallops with black bean salsa and brown rice

Serves 4

⅔ cup instant brown rice (cooked)
    per serving
1 15-oz. can black beans, rinsed
    and drained
1⅓ cups frozen corn, steamed
    and cooled
¼ cup finely chopped red onion
1 small red tomato, chopped
¼ cup loosely packed cilantro
    leaves, chopped

2 Tbsp. fresh lime juice
1 Tbsp. extra-virgin olive oil
½ tsp. salt
½ lb. sea scallops
1 Tbsp. chili powder
1 tsp. sugar
1 Tbsp. canola oil
Cilantro leaves and lime wedges,
    to taste

- Cook brown rice according to package directions.
- In large bowl, make salsa by combining black beans, corn, red onion, tomato, cilantro, lime juice, olive oil, and ¼ teaspoon of the salt. Set aside.
- Rinse scallops with cold running water, then pat dry with paper towels. In medium bowl, mix chili powder, sugar, and remaining ¼ teaspoon salt. Add scallops, tossing to coat.
- In nonstick skillet, heat canola oil over medium-high heat until very hot. Add scallops and cook 3 to 6 minutes until scallops are lightly browned on the outside and turn opaque throughout, turning once.
- Put a bed of brown rice on each plate, followed by scallops, then salsa. Garnish with cilantro and squeeze fresh lime over it, if desired.

545 calories; 32 grams protein; 66 grams carbs (14 grams fiber); 17 grams fat (1 gram saturated)

DESSERTS

Baked balsamic apple or pear

1 medium apple or pear, cut into 1-inch cubes
1 tsp. balsamic vinegar
¼ tsp. ground cardamom

● Preheat oven to 375 degrees. Place cut-up fruit in a small nonstick baking dish. Drizzle with balsamic vinegar and sprinkle with cardamom. Bake 10 to 15 minutes, until fruit is tender.

76 calories; 1 gram protein; 18 grams carbs (4 grams fiber); 0 grams fat

Dark chocolate squares with tea

3 small squares (30 grams) Lindt Excellence Dark Chocolate (i.e., 85% Cocoa)
1 cup brewed decaffeinated herbal tea

153 calories; 3 grams protein; 6 grams carbs (2 grams fiber); 13 grams fat (8 grams saturated)

Lean and Green

Green tea is perhaps the best beverage on the face of the earth, with the possible exception of water. If someone like me had listed all the reputed benefits of green tea—fighting cancer, speeding up metabolism, lowering risk of cardiovascular disease, inhibiting blood clots—in this type of book twenty years ago, you'd have advised me to lay off the acupuncture for a while. Today, it's conceded that green tea has all those benefits, and more—fighting tooth decay, helping your body resist infections . . .

The magic compound in green tea appears to be a polyphenol, similar to the ones in red wine. This one is called EGCG, an antioxidant that has unique potency in green tea, thanks to the fact that the leaves used to make it are steamed instead of fermented. There's nothing wrong with black and oolong teas, which are made from fermented leaves. They just don't have the same health benefits as green tea.

Green tea does have caffeine, but it's a relatively weak dose—about 20 milligrams in a typical tea bag versus 40 milligrams for black tea, 45 for a 12-ounce can of Diet Coke, and 80 for a 5-ounce cup of brewed coffee. Still, the actual dose you get could be higher or lower than that, since tea leaves themselves don't have consistent caffeine levels. Two leaves on the same plant might have different amounts of caffeine.

So while green tea might not be a great choice before bedtime, it's hard to go wrong with it any other time of day.

Lemony fruit, yogurt, and granola parfait

¼ cup fat-free plain yogurt

1 Tbsp. granulated Splenda or stevia (optional)

1 tsp. lemon juice

1 tsp. vanilla extract

¼ cup low-sugar granola (try Bear Naked Fruit and Nut Granola; store.bearnaked.com)

¼ cup fresh or frozen and thawed blueberries

- In medium bowl, mix together yogurt, sweetener, lemon juice, and vanilla.
- Spoon half the granola into the bottom of a glass. Then add half the berries, the yogurt mixture on top of that, the rest of the granola, and finally the remaining berries.

195 calories; 5 grams protein; 28 grams carbs (4 grams fiber); 7 grams fat (1 gram saturated)

High-protein cheesecake

Serves 8

2 cups part-skim ricotta cheese

2 medium eggs

½ cup reduced-fat sour cream

½ cup vanilla whey-protein powder

¼ cup granulated Splenda or stevia

Grated rind and juice of 1 fresh lemon

1 tsp. vanilla extract

- Preheat oven to 375 degrees.
- Put all ingredients in blender, and process until very smooth.
- Spray a 9-inch pie pan with cooking spray. Pour mixture into prepared pan. Place pan on top rack of oven and place a flat pan of water on bottom rack. Bake 30 to 40 minutes. Chill well before serving.

190 calories; 20 grams protein; 7 grams carbs (1 gram fiber); 9 grams fat (5 grams saturated)

SAMPLE FULL-DAY MEAL PLANS

1,700 calories

BREAKFAST: Scrambled egg whites with toast and jam
305 calories; 27 grams protein; 38 grams carbs (10 grams fiber); 5 grams fat (2 grams saturated)

MORNING SNACK: Red pepper and hummus dip
215 calories; 8 grams protein; 19 grams carbs (5 grams fiber); 12 grams fat (1 gram saturated)

LUNCH: Greek salad with chicken
285 calories; 30 grams protein; 12 grams carbs (3 grams fiber); 13 grams fat (3 grams saturated)

MIDAFTERNOON SNACK: Midday shake
233 calories; 26 grams protein; 21 grams carbs (3 grams fiber); 5 grams fat (2 grams saturated)

DINNER: Herb-crusted salmon with asparagus; red wine
560 calories; 50 grams protein; 14 grams carbs (5 grams fiber); 26 grams fat (9 grams saturated); 10 grams alcohol

DESSERT: Baked balsamic apple or pear
76 calories; 1 gram protein; 18 grams carbs (4 grams fiber); 0 grams fat

TOTALS FOR DAY: *1,674 calories; 142 grams protein; 122 grams carbs (30 grams fiber); 61 grams fat (17 grams saturated, 6 grams omega-6, 5 grams omega-3), 10 grams alcohol*

MACRONUTRIENT RATIOS: *Protein: 34 percent; Carbs: 29 percent; Fat: 33 percent; Alcohol: 4 percent*

2,000 calories

BREAKFAST: Oatmeal protein pancakes
355 calories; 39 grams protein; 43 grams carbs (5 grams fiber); 3 grams fat (1 gram saturated)

MORNING SNACK: Multigrain rice cakes topped with Swiss cheese and ham
275 calories; 31 grams protein; 25 grams carbs (1 gram fiber); 6 grams fat (1 gram saturated)

LUNCH: Avocado-tuna salad
372 calories; 25 grams protein; 32 grams carbs (14 grams fiber); 16 grams fat (2 grams saturated)

MIDAFTERNOON SNACK: High-protein yogurt with walnuts
245 calories; 29 grams protein; 14 grams carb (1 gram fiber); 8 grams fat (2 grams saturated)

DINNER: Pork chops with applesauce, steamed spinach, and three-bean salad
590 calories; 53 grams protein; 45 grams carbs (15 grams fiber); 22 grams fat (4 grams saturated)

DESSERT: Dark chocolate squares with tea
153 calories; 3 grams protein; 6 grams carbs (2 grams fiber); 13 grams fat (8 grams saturated)

TOTALS FOR DAY: *1,999 calories; 180 grams protein; 165 grams carbs (38 grams fiber); 68 grams fat (18 grams saturated, 9 grams omega-6, 3 grams omega-3)*

MACRONUTRIENT RATIOS: *Protein: 36 percent; Carbs: 33 percent; Fat: 31 percent*

Omega Plan

If you look closely at the fine print of the two sample meal plans, you'll see that the ratio of omega-6 to omega-3 fats ranges from 6:5 to 9:3 (or 3:1). In the 1,700-calorie plan, the two polyunsaturated fats are nearly equal, while in the 2,000-calorie plan you get more omega-6 fats. There is no agreed-upon ratio in nutrition science. Many believe that the best balance of these two fats is 1:1. Others say that as long as you're not dramatically out of balance—20 grams of omega-6 for every gram of omega-3, for example—you're okay.

As I mentioned previously, I like to get some insurance by taking fish-oil supplements. A typical fish-oil pill has 10 calories, or 1 gram of fat (9 calories) and 1 calorie of something else. About a third of that fat is omega-3, most in the form of the two best types: EPA and DHA. (Trust me, you don't want to know what those stand for. Reading the eighteen syllables would hurt your eyes and fill my computer screen with angry red squiggles from my spell-checker.) So three pills of a generic fish-oil supplement give you 1 gram of omega-3 fats in 30 calories.

It's not a panacea, but it certainly falls into the category of "might help, won't hurt."

PART 3

RESISTANCE IS VITAL

8

Smart Women, Foolish Workouts

CHANCES ARE, when working out with weights in a health club, you do one of two types of programs. If you "do the machines," you go from one muscle-isolating device to the next, with the order of exercises dictated by wherever the gym's designers decided to place the equipment. Or, if you employ a mix of free weights and machines, your workout probably starts off with exercises that emphasize multiple muscle groups—leg presses, lat pulldowns, chest presses—and then shifts to exercises that focus on small muscles. The latter group includes lateral raises for your shoulders, calf raises, biceps curls, and some kind of elbow-straightening exercise for your triceps.

Neither type of workout was designed for you, which brings us to . . .

NEW RULE #18 • Don't do programs designed for someone else's needs

The machine circuit has its origins in marketing. Health clubs could entice members more easily with sleek, shiny machines than with lumps of inert and intimidating iron in the form of barbells and dumbbells. Machines helped them get people in and out of the gyms more efficiently, which is why some entire chains—starting with

Nautilus and culminating with Curves—built their businesses around people using machines in a designated order.

I don't mean this as a blanket smack-down of all exercise machines. Cable machines are terrific. Some other types of machines are useful for research and medical rehabilitation. And some are just fun to use. But most of the machines in your local health club weren't designed for any purpose beyond enriching the manufacturers and club owners.

Benefit to you?

Well, it's better than doing nothing, but there are far better ways to use your time and energy.

The second type of workout is an improvement, but it's still not a routine that was created with your needs in mind. It's an abbreviated version of the workouts popularized by competitive bodybuilders, who train for many hours a week and spend much of that time doing exercises for their smallest muscles. Their goal is to create a physique with dramatic contours and contrasts, and then display it onstage.

What does that have to do with you?

Nothing . . . unless you have dreams of being a competitive bodybuilder. I'm guessing you don't.

So when you choose to do the typical type of program that's suggested for the typical American woman, you're either succumbing to marketing or to the notion that a miniaturized bodybuilding program is ideal for everyone, regardless of her interest in bodybuilding, or lack thereof.

Why are those the only options? *Because health clubs are designed to offer you those options.*

It's not about you; it's about them. Believe me, there's a better way.

OBJECTS IN THE MIRROR . . .

People like me, people who write about exercise and nutrition for a living, are fond of metaphors. We like automobile metaphors when we write about nutrition (food is fuel, in case you haven't heard), and we like building-construction metaphors when we write about strength training ("Build a strong foundation" is sound advice, and can be applied to just about any description of any exercise program).

But the best metaphor is probably electronic:

The typical workout routine suggested for women is like a personal computer that runs on Windows. Windows was built from a platform that was originally designed for an operating system called DOS. Every subsequent version of Windows adds new features to that platform, attempts to address the platform's flaws, and tries to do all this without creating any new security holes through which viruses and worms and spybots and Trojan horses can sneak. But the new Windows is always limited by the basic fact that it's constructed on software that should've been scrapped years ago.

Meanwhile, Apple computers have relatively few problems, mainly because the company's engineers simply started over with a new operating system. And when they realized the limitations of that system, they created a new one, OS-X, which was again built on an entirely new platform and didn't carry over any of the previous system's flaws.

That, in essence, is what Alwyn has done with the programs you'll find in *The New Rules of Lifting for Women*. He starts with three basic assumptions that few exercise scientists and experienced fitness professionals would dispute:

- Each workout should incorporate exercises for all your body's major muscles, since those are the ones that have the most potential to get bigger and stronger, and to shake up your metabolism.
- Absent a medical or sport-specific purpose, exercises that focus on small muscles are usually a waste of time. You can't accomplish anything with a biceps curl that couldn't be achieved with a chin-up or underhand-grip lat pulldown.
- When in doubt, choose exercises that most closely resemble the actions your body was designed to do.

The last point is the one I'm most passionate about. When you do a workout on a randomly configured set of machines, you aren't choosing exercises that mimic your body's movements. You're choosing exercises that support the health club's marketing and layout. And when you do thumbnail versions of bodybuilders' routines, you aren't doing exercises designed to make your body perform better, to make it stronger, faster, and more athletic. A fundamental truth:

The entire point of bodybuilding is to look like something you aren't, to give the appearance of strength and athleticism without actually developing those qualities.

People in my profession like to use the word "training" instead of "lifting" or "working out." Your goal in the gym—or in any type of exercise—is to train your body to do something it doesn't already know how to do, or doesn't do well enough. Thus, if your goal is to lose fat, you don't "work out" to achieve it. You *train* to lose fat.

You teach your body to use more fat for energy while storing less, with the goal of having a leaner body. You do that with the one-two punch of increasing muscle mass while also speeding up your metabolism in every possible way—burning more calories during exercise, burning more calories between workouts, burning more calories while digesting your meals.

If you had to sum up my philosophy in three words, it would probably be "Form follows function." Yes, it's unoriginal, but it works in this context. It's hard to increase the size of your muscles if you aren't actually stronger. And it's hard to speed up your metabolism, with the goal of getting leaner, unless you make your muscles bigger. They may not *look* bigger, as I've said, but you'll get the best results when you add size to the muscle fibers. Thus, you need to get stronger to get leaner. When you get stronger, you also get more athletic, since the best athletes are also the strongest, and the weakest athletes lose. When you're leaner, you'll look stronger and more athletic. Which makes sense, because by that point you *are* stronger and more athletic.

NEW RULE #19 • You don't need to isolate small muscles to make them bigger and stronger

Now let's talk about curls. When you write a book about strength training that includes no specific exercises for small muscles like biceps, triceps, and calves, you owe readers an explanation beyond "because we say so." I understand that the idea of biceps curls and triceps extensions makes intuitive sense—if you want to build those muscles, why wouldn't you work them directly?

But you are working them directly when you do Alwyn's workouts, and the reason you're working them directly is because you're using them the way they were designed to work. The purpose of your biceps is to bend your elbow *while assisting your upper-back muscles* in a pulling motion. A pulling motion can come from overhead, as in climbing, or from out in front of you, as in rowing.

The purpose of your triceps is to straighten your elbow *while assisting your chest and shoulder muscles* in a pushing motion. The push can be overhead, such as putting a box up on a shelf, or out from your torso, like pushing a car that's run out of gas.

Just for a moment, stop and think of all the things your body is designed to do, and thus all the chores your muscles should be able to accomplish. You have to admit that bending and straightening your elbows, as isolated tasks, rank pretty far down the list. Where, outside the gym, are those motions ever separated from the actions of your bigger upper-torso muscles?

And yet the typical woman in the typical gym will spend at least as much time on elbow-bending and elbow-straightening exercises as she does on presses, rows, and pulldowns—the pushing and pulling exercises that mimic the most vital movements your upper body is designed to perform.

I realize this argument is getting long-winded, but I am building to a climactic point: Since your body is designed to use its big and small muscles together, in coordinated movement, doesn't it stand to reason that your body would want to develop those muscles in some systematic, proportional, and coordinated pattern? If you're doing a chest press, for example, is your body going to treat that as a "chest" exercise, and only develop those muscles just because those are the ones you think you're targeting? Of course not; all the muscles designed to accomplish the movement will develop at the same pace.

Thus, a coordinated pushing motion, such as a chest press, will develop your chest, shoulder, and triceps muscles simultaneously and proportionally. A coordinated pulling motion, such as a chin-up or pulldown, will develop your upper back, shoulder, and biceps muscles simultaneously and proportionally. There's no need to isolate those muscles with specific movements; your body knows it needs to increase strength and size in all those muscles to keep them working together synchronously. Why wouldn't it? There's no advantage to developing individual muscles selectively, since strengthening one muscle in isolation creates a proportional weakness in another. Remember, what we're talking about here is training—specifically, *strength* training. Every exercise you do is designed to increase strength, and increasing strength is the key to all the results you want when you lift weights.

Core of Babylon

I FIRST LEARNED the power of the midsection when I was at *Men's Fitness* magazine in the mid-1990s. We were trying to come up with cover lines for our February '94 issue, and realized we had nothing for the "main sell," the big line that draws in readers at the newsstand and sets the tone for the entire issue. Normally, a magazine will use that space to call readers' attention to its biggest, most important story. Fitness magazines typically employ the main sell to spotlight the issue's most exciting diet or workout piece.

But here were the subjects of the features in that month's issue:

- snowboarding
- eating more fruits and vegetables
- jumping rope
- understanding health statistics to tell if a health scare is legitimate or overhyped
- cave diving
- being an involved father

We also had a big sex feature, which was pretty good and which won the magazine its first award from our peers in the publishing industry. But we couldn't make that the main sell for several reasons that aren't worth recounting now.

My point is, we were desperate, and desperate people do desperate things.

We had a two-page column in the back of the magazine called "Spot Training," which highlighted a different muscle group each month and gave readers three exercises to isolate those muscles. (Yes, it hurts to remember that I once did the exact thing I now condemn.) We had never, to the best of my memory, used the column as a main sell. But that month's "Spot Training" just happened to feature the abdominals. So we choked back our professional integrity and went with this cover line: "Awesome Abs: Get a rock-hard stomach in 3 easy steps."

That issue sold better than any in our recent history.

We were hardly the first magazine in history to profit from the promise of better abs, but I think we showed just how low the bar could be set. I mean, even by the standards of two-page, back-of-the-magazine, throwaway columns, that month's Spot Training was pathetic. The exercises themselves were mediocre choices. One of the three was performed incorrectly in the photos. And the model had a worse physique than most of the guys on the magazine's staff. (We weren't exactly impressive in that department. If the editors of *Shape,* our sister magazine, had challenged us to a tug-of-war, the smart money might've been on them.)

Still, when I look back at that episode, the greatest shame I feel is over an aspect of the story that was completely uncontroversial at the time. Each exercise was described as working specific regions of the abdominals—"upper abs," "lower abs," "obliques." I now know that "upper" and "lower" abs simply don't exist, as functional units, even though many people back then believed they did. And the notion that any of the abdominal muscles can or should be worked in isolation from the others is pure fiction.

There's certainly an argument for doing specialized exercises that target the mid-body muscles as a group. Alwyn includes several of them in the programs described in Chapter 10. So, while I'm skeptical about the value of exercises that target other small muscles, like the biceps and deltoids and calves, I have to modify that argument for the muscles in your midsection.

Of course, I have my reasons.

TWISTED FATE

The rectus abdominis, the "six-pack" muscle, is responsible for flexing your torso forward against resistance. (Without a weight to push against, gravity does the trick.) And the obliques, the sets of muscles on the sides of your waist, are designed to twist your upper body and to help you straighten your torso when it's bent to the side.

Stop and think for a moment about when in real life you'd need to perform those actions. Bending forward against some kind of resistance? Outside of the gym, it's hardly ever done. Bending to the side? Again, it's something you see in gyms and dance studios, but in real life it's hardly ever done without also twisting.

Twisting, though, is an important action. Just about everything you do in the office or around the house or yard involves combinations of bends and twists. And every sport, including chess, involves rotation by the middle of your body. Often, those actions are done at top speed in order to generate maximum power.

Think of Maria Sharapova serving a tennis ball 100 mph, or the teenage Michelle Wie driving a golf ball 270 yards off the tee. (I outweigh Wie by 30 pounds, and the only way I could hit a golf ball that far would be downhill. And even then, I'd need a lucky bounce.) Both women are more than six feet tall, with long arms and legs. Add a tennis racquet or golf club and you have extremely long levers whipping the torso around at terrifying speeds. It takes otherworldly talent combined with superb conditioning to twist a human body that hard and that fast without creating some kind of injury to the spine.

Now, having brought up the subject of the spine, I should mention that when I use the word "twist" I'm talking in general about the body's rotational actions. The lumbar spine—the part below your rib cage—doesn't actually twist. Your shoulders turn and your hips rotate, but the bones in your lower back, the vertebrae, aren't supposed to turn independently. They're designed to flex forward and extend backward. So in a ballistic twisting motion, those bones have to have strong muscles and connective tissues holding everything in its designated place.

That's where the rectus abdominis performs what may be its most important role, according to Stuart McGill, Ph.D., professor of spine biomechanics at the University of Waterloo, in Ontario. In his studies and his books, McGill has argued that the rectus abdominis helps hold your torso together during powerful twists. While the obliques are designed to facilitate twisting—that's why the fibers in those muscles run diagonally and horizontally—the rectus seems to prevent *too much* twisting. Its fibers run vertically, up and down. That's the same direction of the fibers on your most prominent lower-back muscles, which we call "spinal erectors" so we don't have to learn any more Latin words than is absolutely necessary. (The Latin name of the muscle is *erector spinae*.) Both sets of muscles, rectus abdominis and spinal erectors, seem to act as brakes to prevent the most extreme twisting motions from pulling your midsection apart.

Which contradicts what we've been told about the muscles in our midsections:

- The crunch is the perfect "ab" exercise, since it builds a visible six-pack.
- A visible six-pack is the ultimate goal of any workout program.
- A bulked-up six-pack will reduce or even prevent lower-back pain.

The reality is different. The basic crunch is, at best, a useless exercise. There are plenty of ways to strengthen your midsection as a unit, including a crunch variation that Alwyn includes in his workouts, without trying to isolate muscles that aren't designed to be isolated. And when it comes to back pain, McGill's research has shown that there's really no connection to midsection strength.

I think there's a better way to look at the goal of abdominal training. It's not to develop the size of the muscles. (I'm sure you're with me on that; I've never met a woman whose goal in the gym was to develop a thicker waistline.) Nor is it to protect your spine *directly*. It's to perform better in everyday activities and specific exercises, and to bolster the integrity of your spine and its connective tissues during the performance of those activities and exercises.

Conversely, putting too much emphasis on abdominal exercises, and using the wrong ones, could actually have a negative effect on your health and posture. Hang with me here as I explain why.

NEW RULE #20 • Every exercise is a "core" exercise

You've heard the term "core training" many times by now. I think it went from "cool, cutting-edge idea" to cliché in record time. You probably know that it's a more sophisticated approach to working your middle body than "ab workouts," which could more accurately be called "bunches of crunches." The "core" includes all the abdominal muscles, along with the muscles in your lower back, hips, pelvis, and upper thighs.

The beauty of core training, as a concept, is that it views your body systemically. Rather than creating artificial separations between "abs" and everything else (not to mention the mostly fictitious "upper abs" and "lower abs"), it starts with the idea that all the muscles involved in moving or protecting your spine and pelvis are united in purpose. Thus, they should be trained as a unit.

Core training, as practiced, pulls in elements from many different disciplines:

- **Yoga,** which helps you master balance and stability through your body's most extreme ranges of motion. You can't have any weak links in the movement chain, so by default you work your midbody area and develop its strength and endurance systemically.
- **Pilates,** which started as rehabilitation exercises for injured dancers and put particular emphasis on what we now call the core. (Joseph Pilates, who created the exercise system, called it the "powerhouse.")
- **Physical therapy,** from which we got the idea of using Swiss balls for targeted exercises. (They're also called stability, balance, or physioballs.)
- **Strength and conditioning,** which provided the idea of using resistance on twisting exercises, including the ones that Alwyn uses in this program.
- **Research into back pain and spine injuries.** McGill has developed and promoted the idea that it's the endurance of the midbody muscles, rather than their strength or flexibility, that helps prevent back pain. You've probably done plank exercises (if you haven't, you'll do them in Alwyn's workouts), which are a good example of an endurance-building drill.

Notice what's missing?

Bodybuilding!

The modern concept of core training either minimizes or eliminates the idea of building a visible six-pack by doing endless series of crunches. Magazine articles still throw a token crunch variation into their core workouts, but it's hard to fault them for clinging to one ghost of workouts past.

So I don't have any dispute with core training, based on the aforementioned disciplines. My only problem is that the concept doesn't go far enough.

DREAD NECK

In the spring of 2006, I heard Bill Hartman lecture at a fitness summit. Bill is a physical therapist and athletic trainer, and consistently ahead of the curve, implementing new ideas years before others in his field have caught on. This time, Bill told us about the concept of "anatomy trains." Roughly speaking, the idea is that your body has a single system of connective tissues that link everything, from head to toe.

We're talking about three kinds of connective tissues:

- *Ligaments,* which connect bones to other bones;
- *Tendons,* which connect muscles to bones or to other connective tissues;
- *Fascia,* which are sheets of tissue that cover muscle bellies and sometimes separate different parts of muscles. The segments of the rectus abdominis, for example, are created by thick bands of fascia, giving the muscle its distinctive resemblance to ice cubes in a tray.

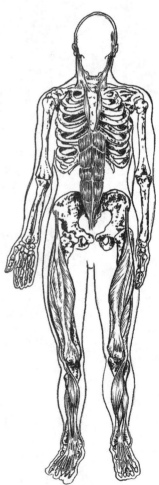

That's the "anatomy" part. "Trains" are the pathways of muscular action that are linked by these connective tissues. And that's where it gets interesting.

In the illustration on this page, you see the rectus abdominis is in the middle of a pathway that starts at the toes, runs up the shins and the quadriceps (the big muscles on the front of your thighs), through the rectus abdominis and the fascia covering your sternum (your breastbone). The path splits as it goes up the sides of your neck, and reconnects on the back of your skull, forming a loop.

This made intuitive sense to me when Bill said it, because it supported an observation I made a few years back while looking at a drawing in an anatomy book. I noticed that the bottom parts of the pectoral muscles—the chest, or "pecs"—were directly connected to the upper parts of the rectus abdominis by a sheath of fascia. You'll never hear a bodybuilder suggest that there's a functional connection between the pecs and the abs—they're two entirely different body parts!—but there it was in that anatomy book, clear as could be.

On the back of your body, the line starts on the bottom of your feet, goes up your calves and hamstrings and spinal erectors, and terminates on the front of your skull, on the ridge of your eyebrows.

Your body also has lines that cross your torso diagonally, as shown on the next page. The one that starts on the inside of your left foot and ankle weaves its way to the outside of your left hip, then crosses the front of your torso (this is why the muscles of your

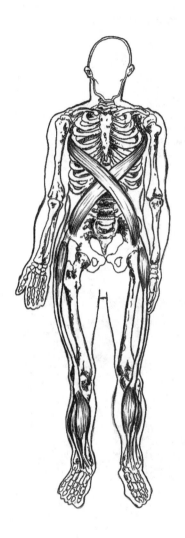

obliques have fibers that go diagonally), wraps behind it, crosses again in your upper back, and ends up on the left-hand side of the base of your skull.

I don't expect you to visualize all that, because my point is a lot simpler: The line of connective tissue that starts at the outside of your left foot ends up at the left side of your skull, almost directly above its origin. But it crosses your torso twice to get there. That leads to an interesting quirk of human physiology—a pain you feel on one side of your upper back could very well have originated on the other side of your lower body. A problem with your foot, like plantar fasciitis, could give you headaches.

Since connective tissues are the train tracks in this theory, muscles are the train stations. That makes the muscles in the middle of your body Grand Central Station, the place where all the lines eventually lead. Some of the lines go straight up the front of your abdominal wall or lower-back muscles, while others crisscross, using your diagonally patterned obliques.

I tell you all this to make two huge points:

First, doing traditional ab exercises on your back on the floor, with your legs bent at the knees and hips, isn't a good use of your time and energy. Whatever benefit you get from "isolating" your rectus abdominis and/or obliques is reduced by the disconnection of the muscles of your middle body from the muscles they're designed to work with.

Second, for women, there's a small but genuine risk of neck pain from doing too many exercises that target your rectus abdominis. (This is the "negative effect on your health and posture" I alluded to several pages back.) And to explain that risk fully, I'll need to give it a section of its own.

ALPHA QUADS

At the start of an exercise program, women tend to be stronger on the front of their thighs than on the back. Trainers use the phrase "quad dominant" to describe this imbalance. Put another way, women's hamstrings tend to be weaker than they should be, in relation to their quadriceps.

The problem is a big one to sports scientists. Female athletes have several times the risk of knee injuries as men, and this strength discrepancy is thought to play a role. Research shows that when the quadriceps are more than a third stronger than the hamstrings, a woman is at greater risk of damaging the ligaments that hold her knees together.

A remarkable study performed at Columbia University and published in 2006 discovered the source of the problem. The researchers looked at male and female soccer players between ages ten and eighteen. The preteen, prepubescent girls were already at high risk of injury, due to the fact their quadriceps were 75 percent stronger than their hamstrings. But the teenage, postpubescent girls had an even bigger problem: their quads were 100 percent stronger than their hamstrings. The strength imbalance actually gets *worse* with time. Their mature hamstrings were stronger than before, but those gains were more than offset by even bigger gains in their quadriceps.

That's the perfect illustration of quad dominance—because they used the muscles more, those muscles got even stronger as their bodies matured, and exacerbated what was already a problem. The boys in the study, by comparison, went the other direction—the older ones had a smaller imbalance than the younger ones. Their bodies had learned to use their hamstrings more effectively.

Hold on to the idea that you, as a physically mature woman, already have a tendency to overuse your quadriceps in relation to muscles on the back of your body. And remember that the rectus abdominis, the six-pack muscle, is intimately connected to those very same quadriceps. Now you know why it's absurd to focus on your rectus abdominis, whether you're doing old-fashioned "ab" training or new-school "core" workouts. It's a muscle that just doesn't need all the love you're willing to offer.

But the real kicker is the risk for neck pain. When your quads are too strong, and your rectus is overworked, the muscles on the front of your body tighten. Tight muscles on the front will stretch out the connective tissues on the back, making them longer and comparatively weaker.

Remember how I said the anatomy train on the front of your body loops around the back of your head? When the connective tissues in that train tighten up, creating stretched-out tissues opposite them, your head starts to tilt forward. It's like having a sling around your head, pulling it down toward your chest. The tighter that sling gets, the more pressure there is on the connective tissues in your upper back. Picture an old lady with a dowager's hump. That's the worst-case scenario of quad dominance, and it could lead to chronic neck pain long before it produces a deformed upper spine.

Having said all that, I don't want to leave you with the idea that if you do a crunch you'll hurt your neck. It's hard to picture the old ladies with the humps doing ab workouts in their youth. I'm just trying to make the point that you never want to exacerbate your body's natural or acquired imbalances. If you're a typical woman, your front-body muscles are already stronger than they should be, compared to the muscles on the back of your body. The goal of Alwyn's programs is to train your body to do what it couldn't do before, and one important part of that training is to improve the relative strength of your upper back, lower back, gluteals, and hamstrings. Everything else will get stronger, too, but the ratio will definitely shift.

A Woman's Place Is in the Weight Room

The first thing you'll notice about Alwyn's workouts, displayed in chart form on the following pages, is that they probably don't look like anything you've seen before. And some of the exercise names will seem foreign—*literally* foreign (Romanian deadlift, Bulgarian split squat . . .).

I promise you this: Even if it's not intuitive, it's still easy to learn the lingo and the workout style. The workouts themselves aren't easy, but at this point in our adventure I hope you don't expect them to be. If you do . . . well, I suggest you reread chapters 1, 2, 3, 8, and 9.

Here's a quick overview of the concepts and techniques that may be new to you.

NUMBER OF WORKOUTS PER WEEK

Three is best. Two will work. One is too few, and any more than three is too much.

STAGES

Alwyn's workouts are divided into seven stages.

Stage 1 is a break-in program with a total of sixteen workouts, plus two special workouts at the end. (I'll explain those when I show you the workout itself.) If you do three workouts a week—which we recommend—you'll finish this stage in six weeks. Then you'd take off for a full week before starting Stage 2.

If you're a true beginner, you can extend this stage, doing twenty-four workouts in eight weeks, following by the two special workouts in the ninth week. Then you'd take a full week off before starting Stage 2.

Stages 2, 3, 4, and 5 each require eight workouts. If you're doing three workouts a week, you'll finish each stage in three weeks. It's up to you if you want to take a week off in between each stage, or wait until you've completed several stages before taking a week off. (I'll explain the rationale for break weeks below.)

Stage 6 is a unique strength-focused program, with the goal of getting you to the point at which you can do a full chin-up without assistance. (I know some of you can already do this; for you, this stage will increase your already impressive strength.) You'll do ten workouts, so at the rate of three per week you'll finish in the fourth week.

This is an optional stage; if you're more interested in fat loss than increasing your strength or muscle size, you can go straight from Stage 5 to Stage 7.

You definitely want to take most or all of a week off following Stage 6.

Stage 7 is dubbed "the Final Cut," which means it's designed for one last assault on whatever body fat you still want to shed. You'll do twelve workouts over four weeks.

That's about six months' worth of workouts if you lift three times a week and do all seven stages. And, of course, the programs could last much longer than that if you choose to do two workouts a week.

ALTERNATING WORKOUTS

Each stage includes two workouts, cleverly titled Workout A and Workout B. (If you've ever read Dr. Seuss, you know that Thing 1 and Thing 2 were already taken.) The exception is Stage 7, the Final Cut, which has a slightly different configuration. I'll explain when we get there.

You'll alternate workouts A and B in every program, so a four-week workout schedule could look like this:

Monday	Tuesday	Wednesday	Thursday	Friday	Saturday	Sunday
Workout A	off	Workout B	off	Workout A	off	off
Workout B	off	Workout A	off	Workout B	off	off
Workout A	off	Workout B	off	Workout A	off	off
Workout B	off	Workout A	off	Workout B	off	off

These are all total-body workouts, which means you'll work all your major muscles every time you're in the gym. (And by "gym," I mean wherever you lift. You should be able to do these workouts at home with slight adjustments, which I'll show in the exercise descriptions in Chapter 11.)

That's why you want to take a full day off between each workout, with no more than three workouts in any seven-day period.

You're welcome to do something active on the days in between your weight workouts. You'll see suggestions and parameters in Chapter 12, "Extra Stuff to Do." For now, I'll just say that your goal in a lifting program is to get the benefits of lifting. Doing extra resistance exercise in between these workouts is counterproductive. Doing intervals, or even some modest endurance exercise, could be beneficial. But it could just as easily interfere with your recovery from the weight workouts. Or you could experience anything in between. There are no rules that apply to every woman, so you have to rely on knowledge of your body and exercise history, along with trial and error, to figure out how much nonlifting activity—if you choose to do any at all—works best for you.

RECOVERY

This is a big topic, since it's really about three different issues:

Recovery between sets and exercises

This is the amount of time you take between each set of each exercise. Alwyn is precise about this, and it's designated in the workout charts you'll see later in this chapter. Rest periods are usually 30, 60, or 90 seconds. Most of the time, you'll rest 30 seconds after high-repetition sets (more than 12 reps per set), 60 seconds after moderate repetitions (8 to 12), and 90 seconds after low-rep sets (6 or fewer). The charts will always tell you what amount of rest Alwyn has in mind.

One question we hear a lot: "What happens if I take less time between sets, so I can get out of the gym faster?" Alwyn's standard response is that it's up to you, of course. But you have to understand you're changing the workout if you change the rest intervals. It's still a workout, and it might be a very good workout, but it's different from the one Alwyn designed.

Recovery between workouts

I mentioned this briefly in the previous section. You always want to give your muscles forty-eight hours to recover before you work them again. That's because, as I've mentioned elsewhere, serious strength training creates microtrauma—tiny tears and strains in your muscles and connective tissues. Your body responds to this minor damage by making your muscles bigger and stronger, thus protecting them against future damage. (That protection mechanism explains why you need to mix up your workouts. Your body's goal is to reach stasis so it can stop making adaptations to the stresses you impose on it. Your goal is to keep imposing new stresses so your body keeps making adaptations.)

Some activities help with recovery by promoting blood flow into the muscles. Certainly, yoga could fall into this category. For some people, a jog or swim or bike ride could serve that purpose. But for others, a jog might simply induce more fatigue into the muscles, so you'd be in worse shape the next time you hit the weights. As I said earlier, I can't predict what will or won't help your recovery, except to say that strenuous resistance exercise will never help you recover from strenuous resistance exercise. That's why you need forty-eight hours between workouts. Sometimes an extra day helps, which is why we suggest a limit of three workouts in any seven-day period.

Recovery between stages

I'd like to make a terrible confession about my own workout programs. This is the third consecutive book in which my coauthor and I have adamantly recommended rest weeks between stages of programs. And I almost never follow this advice. That's because I'm fifty; take two or three vacations a year with my wife and three children; go on several business trips a year; and sometimes take time away from the gym just because the kids are off school and it promotes family harmony if I hang around. It would be harder for me *not* to take weeks off. And because I have so many weeks and partial weeks in which I can't follow a serious training program—probably eight breaks a year, on average—I don't bother scheduling weeks off in my workout schedule. I get weeks off whether I want them or not.

So I want to emphasize that this is the least rigid type of planned recovery. You're free to work with your own schedule, and take a week off earlier or later than the schedule suggests if that works better for you. The only rule is that you should take an occasional week off to give your body a chance to recover fully.

I'm talking about more than your muscles:

- *Connective tissues* have a smaller blood supply than your muscles, and take longer to adapt to strenuous exercise. The extra week away from heavy lifting gives them time to catch up.
- Your *nervous system* gets fatigued along with your muscles, tendons, and ligaments. This is something exercise scientists have only recently begun exploring, so there aren't yet firm guidelines. But strength coaches like Alwyn and longtime lifters like me understand that sometimes you have bad days in the gym, even though your muscles have had plenty of time to recover. We often call that "neural fatigue," which is a fancy way of saying the body is willing but the brain has other ideas.
- *Bones* also need time to make adaptations. The strain of lifting causes your body to put down new collagen fibers. Those fibers eventually harden into functional bone tissue. It's a months-long process, so by design the adaptation of your bones to heavy lifting lags behind the recovery of your connective tissues, which itself lags behind the recovery of your muscles. And the recovery of your nervous system is a wild card. The best insurance that everything recovers and rebuilds itself is to take a week off from time to time.

ALTERNATING SETS

When you look at the workout charts, you'll notice that each exercise has a letter preceding it. The first exercise is labeled either A or A1. Most of the time, the second exercise is B1, followed by B2. (Sometimes there's also a B3 or even a B4.) This is the most potentially confusing part of the workout system, and I'm going to explain it as carefully as I can. (In other words, if you already understand why exercises are labeled this way, you'll want to skip this section.)

If an exercise is presented with simply a letter (A) that means it's a stand-alone exercise, and you do it in "straight sets"—you do the designated sets with the designated amount of rest following each of them.

If the exercises have a letter and a number (B1, B2), then you're going to do them as alternating sets. The technique is simple. You do the first exercise (B1, say), rest for the designated time, do the second exercise (B2), rest for the designated time, and repeat until you've done all the required sets of both exercises.

Let's look at an example, from Stage 1:

Exercise		Sets	Reps	Rest (seconds)
Alternating sets				
B1	Push-up	2	12	60
B2	Seated row	2	12	60

As I said, this is straightforward. You do a set of twelve push-ups (you'll see several variations starting on page 188 that allow for women of all strength levels to complete the repetitions), rest 60 seconds, do a set of twelve seated rows, rest, and repeat.

Here's why Alwyn designs his workouts this way:

First, let's imagine that you were doing these exercises the traditional way. You'd do a set of push-ups, which takes you about 30 seconds. You rest 60 seconds, do the next set of push-ups, then rest another 60 seconds.

You're doing 30 seconds of exercise every 90 seconds, which is an efficient way to train. And in this context, I'm not using "efficient" as a pejorative. I mean you're making productive use of your time.

But now let's see what happens when you do alternating sets of two different exercises, which work different muscle groups:

Push-ups, set 1: 30 seconds
Rest: 60 seconds
Rows, set 1: 30 seconds
Rest: 60 seconds
Push-ups, set 2: 30 seconds
Rest: 60 seconds
Rows, set 2: 30 seconds
Rest: 60 seconds

In this system, you're still using your time efficiently—30 seconds of exercise every 90 seconds. But now you're allowing the muscles you use in the individual exercises to recover for 150 seconds between sets, instead of 60. That's two and a half minutes of recovery, with only 30 seconds of that time exercising unrelated muscle groups.

When you get down on the floor for your second set of push-ups, you're certainly going to be stronger in this scenario than you would've been in the first. You can work with more intensity and/or do a more challenging variation of the exercise, and thus develop more strength and muscle size.

If the workout calls for a B3 and/or B4, the technique is the same. Do the exercises in sequence, with the designated rest periods in between, and repeat as many times as required.

WARMING UP

A good warm-up serves three purposes:

- It raises the temperature in the muscles you're about to work and starts the flow of adrenaline, which stimulates your nervous system and allows more blood to reach your muscles.
- It gets muscles, joints, and nerves ready for the specific actions you want them to perform.
- It accomplishes the first two goals without depleting a significant amount of the energy you'll need for the actual workout.

There's no such thing as a "perfect" warm-up technique that applies to everyone. On a hot summer day, just walking from your car to the gym might be enough to raise your core temperature, allowing you to skip that first step. On a cold day, you may need to spend ten to fifteen minutes on an exercise bike or treadmill to get that same effect.

The same goes for morning versus afternoon or evening exercise. Mornings require longer, more gradual warm-ups, whereas your temperature and heart rate will naturally be a bit higher and faster if you work out at lunch or after work.

Once you're satisfied with your general warm-up—that is, your core temperature and heart rate are elevated a bit, in your estimation (you certainly don't have to measure this)—you can do what I call a semi-specific warm-up. These are exercises that are like the ones you'll do in an actual workout, but aren't meant to function as specific preparation for those exercises. The goal is to move muscles and joints through full ranges of motion.

If I can return to the computer analogy I used in Chapter 8, the general warm-up is like turning on your body's power switch. This semi-specific warm-up is like firing up the software you're going to use. The specific warm-up, which I'll describe in a moment, is akin to opening or creating the files or documents you're going to work on. And then the workout is the actual data you put into those files or documents.

You can accomplish a semi-specific warm-up without any prescribed routine (why get specific about a semi-specific warm-up?). Just do some simple, nonstrenuous exercises that mimic exercises you'll do in Alwyn's programs.

If you want a sample routine, try these four exercises:

SQUAT TO STAND

➤ Stand with your feet shoulder-width apart. Bend and grab your toes. With your arms straight and inside your knees, squat down. Keep your lower back flat and pull your shoulder blades together as you push your chest forward. Now stand and straighten your legs, feeling a good stretch in your hamstrings. Hold for 1 or 2 seconds, then squat again. *Do 5 to 8 repetitions.*

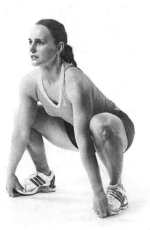 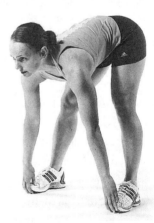

LATERAL LUNGE

➤ Stand with your feet shoulder-width apart, toes pointed straight ahead, and hands together in front of your chest. Lunge to your right, sinking as low as you can while keeping your lower back in its naturally arched position. (Don't let your back round forward, in other words.) Hold for 1 or 2 seconds, then return to the starting position, and lunge to your left. *Do 5 lunges to each side.*

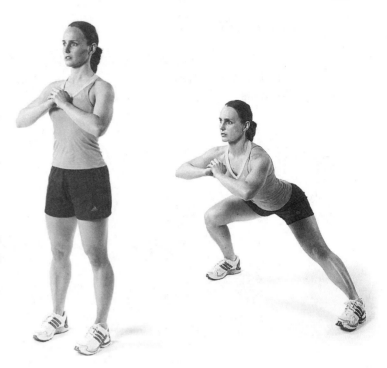

REVERSE LUNGE WITH TWIST AND OVERHEAD REACH

➤ Stand with your feet hip-width apart, hands at your sides. Lunge back with your right leg, while turning your head and shoulders to the left and reaching over your head with your right arm. Hold for 1 second. Return to the starting position, then lunge backward with your left leg, turning your shoulders to the right and reaching overhead with your left arm. *Do 5 lunges with each leg.*

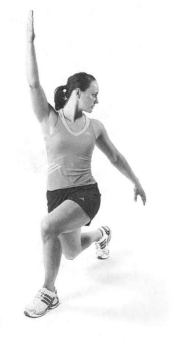

INCHWORM

➤ Stand with your feet together. Bend forward and place your hands on the floor. Walk your hands out until you're in a push-up position, with your body forming a straight line from neck to ankles. Now walk your feet up to your hands. *Do 5 to 8 repetitions.*

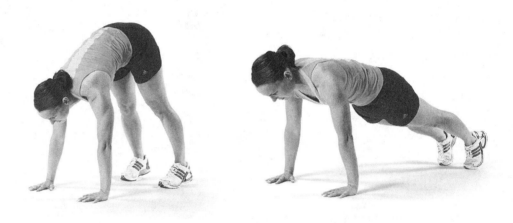

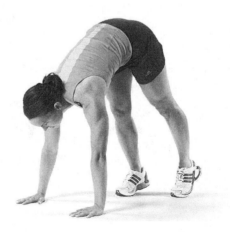

Now comes the most important part of the warm-up: preparing your body for the specific exercises you're about to perform. If the first exercise in your workout is squats, for example, you want to do at least a set or two to get your body ready. How many warm-up sets you do depends on whether the workout calls for light, medium, or heavy weights:

Light (more than 12 repetitions per set)

Do one warm-up set of 8 repetitions with about two-thirds of the weight you'll be using in your first set. In Stage 1, you'll be starting each workout with either squats or deadlifts. Your initial workouts call for two sets of 15 repetitions of those exercises. Since you aren't likely to use a lot of weight, you could simply warm up using your body weight on the squats, and perhaps an empty barbell for the deadlifts. I don't like to prescribe specific starting weights for any exercise (as I'll explain in the next section), so this is really up to you. The key is to practice the exercise through the full range of motion before doing the "work" sets, the ones listed in the workout charts.

Medium (8 to 12 repetitions per set)

Do two warm-up sets:

- 5 to 8 reps with about 50 percent of the weight you'll use in your first set
- 4 to 6 reps with about 75 percent of the first-set weight

Heavy (fewer than 8 repetitions per set)

Do three warm-up sets:

- 5 to 6 reps with about 50 percent of the weight you'll use in your first set
- 3 to 4 reps with about 75 percent of the first-set weight
- 2 to 3 reps with about 90 percent of the first-set weight

This is for the first exercise in each workout. Should you do warm-ups for subsequent exercises? That's up to you. I don't know of any research that answers the question. In my own workouts, I'll do warm-up sets for any exercise calling for heavy weights with muscles I haven't already used in the workout. So if the first exercise is squats or deadlifts (lower body) and the next exercise is bench presses or rows (upper body), and the weights are heavy (fewer than 8 repetitions), I recommend doing a warm-up set or two for that subsequent exercise.

I wish I could be more specific, but the truth is that additional warm-up sets could have a negative effect if they sap some of the energy you need to complete the workout. But at the same time, your muscles, joints, and nerves will always perform better with proper preparation. So the best advice I can offer is to preserve energy by minimizing warm-ups before doing high-repetition sets. When the workout calls for low reps and heavy weights, go for safety and performance by warming up specifically for the first two or three exercises in that routine, and use your own judgment on subsequent exercises.

If you feel that you need a specific warm-up for any exercise, at any point in your routine, you probably do.

HOW MUCH WEIGHT TO USE?

You'd think this would be a straightforward question. It isn't. I hear this question a lot, and from women and men in just about equal numbers. There are three variations on the question:

✴ **How do I select a weight to use for an exercise I've never done before?**
If you were a guy, I'd say this: "Pick the weight you can think you can use for the number of repetitions the workout requires, and then deduct 25 percent." For women, I'm tempted to say that opposite—"Whatever you think you can use, the actual amount is probably higher."

But that would be glib, not to mention useless, especially if you've never lifted before and have no idea where to start.

So let's make it simpler:

Start light, and try to increase the weight you use every time you do that workout.

If using nothing but your own body weight is an option—as it is with squats, lunges, Swiss-ball crunches, and many others—start with that.

If you're given a number of variations of increasing difficulty—we offer several push-up variations, for example—start with the easiest and work your way toward the hardest.

Remember, this is a six-month program, more or less. There's plenty of time for trial and error. If you choose a weight that's too easy for one workout, increase it in the next by the smallest possible increment, and then keep increasing it throughout the program.

Having said that, I don't want you to start with the 1-pound Barbie weights and, over the course of eight weeks, advance all the way up to the 8-pound Barbie weights. Lifting weights should always feel like *lifting weights*. If it doesn't feel like exercise, it's not doing what you want it to do.

* **Do I use the same weight for every set of an exercise in a workout, or do I use slightly more weight each set?**

It's up to you. Let's say you're doing three sets of 10 repetitions of lat pulldowns, and you've chosen not to do any warm-up sets for this specific exercise. (It'll never come first in your workouts, so you'll always have this choice.) You do the first set with 30 pounds, and you know by the third repetition that this weight is far too light.

Your best strategy: Finish the set, then increase the weight to 40 pounds for the second set. If that's still too easy, increase it for the third set, perhaps to 45 pounds. (Your gym probably has removable plates that allow you to go up by 2.5 or 5 pounds, rather than the standard 10-pound increases required by the machine's fixed plates.) If even that's too light, then make a note on your training log (if you don't know what that is, I'll explain in the next section), and use more weight the next time you do that workout.

* **Should I choose a weight that allows me to go to failure, or should I stop short of that point?**

You're excused for not knowing that the "failure/short-of-failure" debate is the exercise-science equivalent of "form/content." If you had no idea that a debate even exists, trust me, you're better off. And if you don't even know what the heck I'm talking about . . . well, let's start there.

In the previous example, your workout called for three sets of 10 repetitions of lat pulldowns. That leaves open the question of how difficult those repetitions should be. Should the tenth repetition be so difficult that you can barely complete it, and at the end of three sets your arms shake uncontrollably and you'd rather scrub the showers in your gym's locker room than do another set?

No.

I don't think you ever need to push yourself that far in the weight room. Your goal should be to make your sets challenging—they should feel like work, and the deeper you get into the six-month program, the harder they should feel. But you never need to get to the point at which the last repetition of a set is the last rep your body could possibly perform.

Not intentionally, that is.

There will certainly be times in which you get to the ninth rep of a 10-rep set and realize you can't possibly do the tenth and final one. That's fine—in fact, it's more than fine; it's proof that you're challenging yourself. Good for you.

But you never need to try to hit that point of total muscular exhaustion on any set, and you *absolutely never* need to extend a set past the designated numbers of repetitions just so your muscles get to that point of momentary failure.

I should also note here, as an aside to those of you who're new to lifting, that everything I've just described is a moving target. You're stronger on some days than you are on others, just as you sometimes feel as if you have more energy on some days and less on others. If you really push yourself on one exercise, you may feel slightly weaker on the next one.

So if you don't go to the limit, how do you know what to shoot for?

The first time you do a new workout, you want to choose a weight that allows you to stop a set feeling as if you could easily do two or three more repetitions. So if it calls for 10 reps, you want to select a weight that you think you could do as many as twelve or thirteen times. This will never be something you can guess precisely, as I said. But that's your goal. The next time you do that workout, you want to use more weight on each exercise, so you would choose one that you think you could do at least ten times, but certainly not twelve or more.

The third time through the workout, you want to select a weight that you're pretty sure you can do ten times, but no more. And the fourth time, you'd pick a weight that you may or may not be able to do ten times. If you stop short of ten, that's okay—it's your last time with that particular exercise for that number of repetitions, so you want to push your limits.

But that doesn't mean going to total muscular failure on any set of any exercise. You simply go to the last rep you can do with good form, and stop there. If you don't think you can finish the next repetition, don't start it.

KEEPING A TRAINING LOG

This is an absolute, inviolable rule: You must keep track of each workout. I've included a blank training log on page 137. You can photocopy that, and fill in the exercises, sets, and reps. Or you can go to newrulesoflifting.com and download a blank log page.

New Rules of Lifting for Women
Stage:
Workout:

Exercise	Sets	Reps	Set 1	Set 2	Set 3	Set 4	Rest
Workout 1							
Workout 2							
Workout 3							
Workout 4							
Workout 1							
Workout 2							
Workout 3							
Workout 4							
Workout 1							
Workout 2							
Workout 3							
Workout 4							
Workout 1							
Workout 2							
Workout 3							
Workout 4							
Workout 1							
Workout 2							
Workout 3							
Workout 4							
Workout 1							
Workout 2							
Workout 3							
Workout 4							

Notes: _____

_____

Using one is pretty simple. Once you've photocopied or downloaded the page and filled out the information you need, just attach it to a clipboard, take it to the gym, and fill in the weight you use and repetitions you complete for each set of each exercise.

Here's an example of how you might record a workout:

New Rules of Lifting for Women
Stage *1*
Workout *A*

Exercise	Sets	Reps	Set 1	Set 2	Set 3	Set 4	Rest
A: Squat							
Workout 1	2	15	BW/15	10/15			60
Workout 2							
Workout 3							
Workout 4							
Alternating sets							
B1: Push-up—variation #2 (45 degrees)							
Workout 1	2	15	14	12			60
Workout 2							
Workout 3							
Workout 4							
B2: Seated row							
Workout 1	2	15	30/15	35/15			60
Workout 2							
Workout 3							

The "BW" notation for squats is shorthand for "body weight," meaning you didn't use any extra weights. The "15" following that means you did all 15 repetitions required by the workout. For the next set, you chose to use 10 pounds, and still got all 15.

Conversely, when you did push-ups, you chose a variation that allowed you to do 14 reps in the first set, and just 12 in the second. That's the way it goes with body-weight exercises. We offer several push-up variations, each of which requires progressively more strength to perform, but ultimately a body-weight exercise will never give you the same versatility you'll find at the dumbbell rack. You can't lop off parts of your body to make yourself heavier or lighter in 5-pound increments, and there are limited ways to play the angles. So your best strategy is to find the variation that allows you to get closest to the target repetitions. As you get stronger in future workouts, you should hit 15 easily, and will soon be ready to move up to a more challenging variation.

THE WORKOUTS

Stage 1

You'll note, as soon as you look at the workout chart, that each exercise shows four different combinations of sets and reps. You'll go from 15 reps per set to 12, 10, and then 8. That guarantees you'll be using heavier weights and doing more challenging variations of exercises like push-ups.

The chart shows you doing two workouts at each level—two workouts with 15 reps, two with 12, etc. But if you're a beginner, or someone who's doing these particular exercises for the first time, feel free to add a third workout at each level. That means you'll do twenty-four workouts in Stage 1, instead of sixteen, and spend eight weeks at this stage. It is absolutely fine to take it slowly, particularly if you feel you need several workouts to get comfortable with the exercises and techniques.

But whether you do each level two or three times, the same rule applies. Your goal is to use more weight in every exercise, in every workout. If the exercise is done with body weight, like push-ups, you want to increase your performance from workout to workout—more repetitions of a variation, then a more difficult variation, then more repetitions of that, and so on.

Sometimes it'll be impractical to move up that steadily. With dumbbells, for example, the increments are too large to allow for that kind of progress. Some gyms won't offer any dumbbell weights that aren't divisible by five, so moving up from 5 to 10 implies a doubling in strength, and from 10 to 15 means another 50 percent jump. You'll get stronger on Alwyn's programs, but nobody increases their strength *that* fast.

Workout A		Sets	Reps	Rest (seconds)
Exercise				
A	Squat (page 157)			
	Workouts 1, 2	2	15	60
	Workouts 3, 4	2	12	60
	Workouts 5, 6	3	10	60
	Workouts 7, 8	3	8	60
Alternating sets				
B1	Push-up (page 191)			
	Workouts 1, 2	2	15	60
	Workouts 3, 4	2	12	60
	Workouts 5, 6	3	10	60
	Workouts 7, 8	3	8	60
B2	Seated row (page 202)			
	Workouts 1, 2	2	15	60
	Workouts 3, 4	2	12	60
	Workouts 5, 6	3	10	60
	Workouts 7, 8	3	8	60
Alternating sets				
C1	Step-up (page 171)			
	Workouts 1, 2	2	15	60
	Workouts 3, 4	2	12	60
	Workouts 5, 6	3	10	60
	Workouts 7, 8	3	8	60
C2	Prone jackknife (page 215)			
	Workouts 1, 2	2	8	60
	Workouts 3, 4	2	10	60
	Workouts 5, 6	3	12	60
	Workouts 7, 8	3	15	60

Workout B

Exercise		Sets	Reps	Rest (seconds)
A	Deadlift (page 164)			
	Workouts 1, 2	2	15	60
	Workouts 3, 4	2	12	60
	Workouts 5, 6	3	10	60
	Workouts 7, 8	3	8	60
Alternating sets				
B1	Dumbbell shoulder press (page 185)			
	Workouts 1, 2	2	15	60
	Workouts 3, 4	2	12	60
	Workouts 5, 6	3	10	60
	Workouts 7, 8	3	8	60
B2	Wide-grip lat pulldown (page 199)			
	Workouts 1, 2	2	15	60
	Workouts 3, 4	2	12	60
	Workouts 5, 6	3	10	60
	Workouts 7, 8	3	8	60
Alternating sets				
C1	Lunge (page 173)			
	Workouts 1, 2	2	15	60
	Workouts 3, 4	2	12	60
	Workouts 5, 6	3	10	60
	Workouts 7, 8	3	8	60
C2	Swiss-ball crunch (page 218)			
	Workouts 1, 2	2	8	60
	Workouts 3, 4	2	10	60
	Workouts 5, 6	3	12	60
	Workouts 7, 8	3	15	60

Special workouts: After you finish your final workouts, do two bonus workouts. For each exercise, use the same weights you used in your very first workout. But instead of stopping at 15 repetitions—or however many you completed—do as many as you can. (On the following charts, I've abbreviated this as "AMRAP," for "as many reps as possible.") This should give you a pretty good approximation of how much progress you've made in just six to eight weeks.

Special Workout A

Exercise		Sets	Reps	Rest (seconds)
A	Squat (page 157)	1	AMRAP	60
B	Push-up (page 191)	1	AMRAP	60
C	Seated row (page 202)	1	AMRAP	60
D	Step-up (page 171)	1	AMRAP	60
E	Prone jackknife (page 215)	1	AMRAP	60

Special Workout B

Exercise		Sets	Reps	Rest (seconds)
A	Deadlift (page 164)	1	AMRAP	60
B	Dumbbell shoulder press (page 185)	1	AMRAP	60
C	Wide-grip lat pulldown (page 199)	1	AMRAP	60
D	Lunge (page 173)	1	AMRAP	60
E	Swiss-ball crunch (page 218)	1	AMRAP	60

Stage 2

Do each workout four times.

Workout A				
Exercise		**Sets**	**Reps**	**Rest (seconds)**
A	Front squat/push press (page 180)	2	10	75
Alternating sets				
B1	Step-up (page 171)	2	10	75
B2	Dumbbell one-point row (page 205)	2	10	75
Alternating sets				
C1	Static lunge, rear foot elevated (page 175)	2	10	75
C2	Push-up (page 191)	2	10	75

Exercise		**Sets**	**Reps**	**Rest (seconds)**
Alternating sets				
D1	Plank (page 213)	2	60 seconds*	75
D2	Cable horizontal wood chop (page 225)	2	10	75

* On the plank, you want to hold whichever variation you choose for 60 seconds. If you can't hold even the easiest variation for that long, then you need to use this technique: Hold as long as you can (30 seconds, say). Then rest that exact same amount of time (30 seconds), then do the final 30 seconds of the set. Now rest 60 seconds, and do a set of wood chops. Rest 60 seconds, and repeat the plank drill.

Workout B				
Exercise		**Sets**	**Reps**	**Rest (seconds)**
A	Wide-grip deadlift from box (page 166)	2	10	75
B1	Bulgarian split squat (page 176)	2	10	75
B2	Underhand-grip lat pulldown (page 200)	2	10	75
C1	Reverse lunge from box with forward reach (page 177)	2	10	75
C2	Dumbbell prone Cuban snatch (page 207)	2	10	75
D1	Swiss-ball crunch (page 218)	2	10	75
D2	Reverse crunch (page 216)	2	10	75
D3	Lateral flexion (pages 221–24)*	2	10	75
E	Prone cobra (page 227)	2	60–90 seconds**	75
Interval training				
15 minutes				
1 minute hard/2 minutes recovery				
*Choose one. **The idea here is the same as described earlier for the plank.				

A few words about interval training

Interval training is a lot like strength training, in that the goal is to give your body a stimulus from which it needs some time to recover. That means you'll burn more calories—especially fat calories—in the hours after you're finished. But it's also like strength training in this respect: Most people don't get all the benefits it has to offer.

Two typical mistakes:

1. An aggressive exerciser will go all-out the first time she tries it, and find the experience so miserable that she never wants to do it again.
2. A more timid exerciser will do it at the exact same intensity every time. After the first few weeks, her body has made all the adaptations it's going to make, and after that she's just going through the motions.

A better approach is to go slowly at first, build up a base of anaerobic fitness, and then gradually push yourself into doing tougher intervals—with greater benefits. To give an example of what I mean, let's use a stationary bike, since it has numerical progressions that are easy to remember.

First interval session
Warm-up: 3 minutes level 1, 2 minutes level 2
Interval 1: 1 minute level 4
Recovery 1: 2 minutes level 1
Interval 2: 1 minute level 4
Recovery 2: 2 minutes level 1
Interval 3: 1 minute level 4
Recovery 3: 2 minutes level 1

That's fourteen minutes, which is plenty for the first time.

Second interval session
Warm-up: 1 minute level 1, 2 minutes level 2
Interval 1: 1 minute level 4
Recovery 1: 2 minutes level 1
Interval 2: 1 minute level 5
Recovery 2: 2 minutes level 1
Interval 3: 1 minute level 5
Recovery 3: 2 minutes level 1
Interval 4: 1 minute level 5
Recovery 4: 2 minutes level 1

That's fifteen minutes, with a shorter warm-up and three minutes at a higher level of intensity than you approached in the first session.

Third interval session
Warm-up: 1 minute level 1, 2 minutes level 2
Interval 1: 1 minute level 4
Recovery 1: 2 minutes level 1
Interval 2: 1 minute level 5
Recovery 2: 2 minutes level 1

Interval 3: 1 minute level 6
Recovery 3: 2 minutes level 1
Interval 4: 1 minute level 6
Recovery 4: 2 minutes level 1

This is still more work than you did in the second session, but you're giving your body time to adjust. Ideally, you should feel as if you're holding back at this point—you know your body can do more, but you're not yet ready to push your limits.

Fourth interval session
Warm-up: 1 minute level 1, 2 minutes level 2
Interval 1: 1 minute level 5
Recovery 1: 2 minutes level 1
Interval 2: 1 minute level 6
Recovery 2: 2 minutes level 1
Interval 3: 1 minute level 7
Recovery 3: 2 minutes level 1
Interval 4: 1 minute level 7
Recovery 4: 2 minutes level 1

Again, you know you could go harder, but not *a lot* harder. So, after four sessions, you've built up to the point where you're testing yourself, but you're still not at your limits.

You can do intervals on foot or on a bike outdoors, or with any type of machine indoors. The key is steady, gradual improvement—a little more work each time, rather than big leaps of effort and intensity that leave you feeling beaten down, rather than worked up.

If you're not using a gym machine, you can use several ways to judge how hard you're working:

- Heart-rate monitor. If you know how fast your heart is pumping, you can push yourself harder over time. As a bonus, you can also see how fast your heart recovers from a tough interval, which is a good measure of heart health.
- Pedometer. If you're taking more steps during your one-minute intervals, you're probably going faster.
- Distance. Traveling farther on your intervals is another sign of increasing speed, and thus increasing effort.

Stage 3

Same as Stage 2—eight total workouts.

Workout A		Sets	Reps	Rest (seconds)
Exercise				
A	One-armed dumbbell snatch (page 183)	3	6	105
Alternating sets				
B1	Dumbell single-leg Romanian deadlift (page 170)	3	6	105
B2	Barbell bent-over row (page 203)	3	6	105
Alternating sets				
C1	Dumbbell single-arm overhead squat (page 162)	3	6	105
C2	Dumbbell incline bench press (page 195)	3	6	105
Alternating sets				
D1	Plank (page 213)	3	90 seconds	105
D2	Reverse wood chop (page 226)	3	6	105
Body-weight matrix				
24 squats				
12 lunges (each leg)				
12 lunge jumps (each leg)				
24 squat jumps				
Time yourself on the matrix. Rest twice as long as it took you to perform the exercises, and repeat.				

Workout B

Exercise		Sets	Reps	Rest (seconds)
A	Barbell Romanian deadlift/bent-over row (page 182)	3	6	105
Alternating sets				
B1	Partial single-leg squat (page 160)	3	6	105
B2	Wide-grip lat pulldown (page 199)	3	6	105
Alternating sets				
C1	Back extension (page 227)	3	6	105
C2	YTWL (page 208)	3	6	105
Alternating sets (abdominal circuit)				
D1	Swiss-ball crunch (page 218)	3	6	105
D2	Hip flexion (pages 215–17)*	3	6	105
D3	Lateral flexion (pages 221–24)*	3	6	105
E	Prone cobra (page 227)	3	90 seconds	105
Interval training				
15 minutes 1 minute hard/2 minutes recovery **Choose one.				

Intervals: Your goal is the same as it was in Stage 2—gradual improvement. But first, take a step back. Do one fewer interval than you did in the final three sessions of Stage 2, so your workout is twelve minutes, rather than fifteen, and don't go any harder than you did in Stage 2. (If you peaked at Level 7 on a stationary bike, don't go up to Level 8 yet.)

For the second, third, and fourth sessions, go back to fifteen minutes, and gradually move up to higher intensity.

Stage 4

Again, do each workout four times, for a total of eight workouts.

Workout A

Exercise		Sets	Reps	Rest (seconds)
A	Front squat/push press (page 180)	2–3	8	90
Alternating sets				
B1	Step-up (page 171)	2–3	8	90
B2	Dumbbell one-point row (page 205)	2–3	8	90

Alternating sets				
C1	Static lunge, rear foot elevated (page 175)	2–3	8	90
C2	Push-up (page 191)	2–3	8	90
Alternating sets				
D1	Plank (page 213)	2–3	120 seconds	90
D2	Cable horizontal wood chop (page 225)	2–3	8	90

Workout B				
Exercise		**Sets**	**Reps**	**Rest (seconds)**
A	Wide-grip deadlift from box (page 166)	2–3	8	90
Alternating sets				
B1	Bulgarian split squat (page 176)	2–3	8	90
B2	Underhand-grip lat pulldown (page 200)	2–3	8	90
Alternating sets				
C1	Reverse lunge from box with forward reach (page 177)	2–3	8	90
C2	Dumbbell prone Cuban snatch (page 207)	2–3	8	90
Alternating sets (abdominal circuit)				
D1	Swiss-ball crunch (page 218)	2–3	8	90
D2	Reverse crunch (page 216)	2–3	8	90
D3	Lateral flexion (pages 221–24)*	2–3	8	90
E	Prone cobra (page 227)	2–3	120 seconds	90
Interval training				
15 minutes 1 minute hard/2 minutes recovery *Choose one.				

Intervals: Use the same strategy you used in Stage 3—take a step back in the first session, then take small steps forward in the next three.

Stage 5

Do each workout four times, for a total of eight workouts.

Workout A		Sets	Reps	Rest (seconds)
Exercise				
A	One-armed dumbbell snatch (page 183)	3–4	4	120
Alternating sets				
B1	Dumbbell single-leg Romanian deadlift (page 170)	3–4	4	120
B2	Barbell bent-over row (page 203)	3–4	4	120
Alternating sets				
C1	Dumbbell single-arm overhead squat (page 162)	3–4	4	120
C2	Dumbbell incline bench press (page 195)	3–4	4	120
Alternating sets				
D1	Plank (page 213)	3	120 seconds	120
D2	Reverse wood chop (page 226)	3	4	120
Body-weight matrix				
24 squats				
12 lunges (each leg)				
12 lunge jumps (each leg)				
24 squat jumps				
Rest twice as long as it took you to perform the exercises, and repeat.				

Workout B		Sets	Reps	Rest (seconds)
Exercise				
A	Barbell Romanian deadlift/bent-over row (page 182)	3–4	4	120
Alternating sets				
B1	Partial single-leg squat (page 160)	3–4	4	120
B2	Wide-grip lat pulldown (page 199)	3–4	4	120
Alternating sets				
C1	Back extension (page 227)	3–4	4	120
C2	YTWL (page 208)	3–4	4	120
Alternating sets (abdominal circuit)				
D1	Swiss-ball crunch (page 218)	3–4	4	120
D2	Hip flexion (pages 215–17)*	3–4	4	120
D3	Lateral flexion (pages 221–24)*	3–4	4	120
E	Prone cobra (page 227)	3	120 seconds	120
Interval training				
15 minutes 1 minute hard/2 minutes recovery *Choose one.				

Intervals: Same strategy as stages 3 and 4.

Stage 6

These strength-focused workouts depart from the previous stages in several important ways. The most noticeable departure is the first exercise in Workout A: negative chin-ups. You'll see that instead of doing repetitions the traditional way, you'll start with your chin over the bar, and then lower yourself as slowly as possible. More specific instructions are embedded in the workout chart, along with modifications for the other exercises.

Your goal here is to develop more strength relative to your body weight. That's why you'll focus on chin-ups and push-ups in Workout A.

Do each workout five times, for a total of ten workouts.

Earlier in this chapter, I noted that this stage is optional—if you're more interested in rapid fat loss than developing strength (and the ability to do an unassisted chin-up with your body weight), you can go straight to Stage 7.

Final note: You'll see the acronym AMRAP in the charts; it means, "as many reps as possible."

Workout A				
Exercise		**Sets**	**Reps**	**Rest (seconds)**
A	Negative chin-up (page 198)	3	1*	60
B	Underhand-grip lat pulldown †			
	Workout 1	10	2	60
	Workout 2	10	2	45
	Workout 3	10	2	30
	Workout 4	10	2	15
	Workout 5	1	AMRAP	n/a
Alternating sets				
C1	Barbell split squat (page 174)			
	Workout 1	2	10	60
	Workout 2	2	8	60
	Workout 3	3	6	60
	Workout 4	3	4	60
	Workout 5	2	10‡	60
C2	Push-up (page 191)**			
	Workout 1	2	10	60
	Workout 2	2	8	60
	Workout 3	3	6	60
	Workout 4	3	4	60
	Workout 5	2	AMRAP	60

* Lower yourself as slowly as possible. Once you can extend this negative chin-up to 20 seconds, you need to add some extra weight to make it harder. Start with 5 pounds. If you work out in a gym, you can probably find a special belt with a chain that allows you to hang a weight plate or dumbbell from your waist. Or, if you work out at home, you can put a 5-pound weight into a backpack and wear that.

† Perform each repetition this way:
1. Pull the bar down as fast as you can.
2. Pause 1 second.
Take 4 seconds to return the weight to the starting position.

‡ Use the same weight in workouts 2 and 5, but do 2 more reps per set in Workout 5 (10 instead of 8).

** This time, do the same push-up variation each workout, but with this modification: In each workout, make it more difficult by either adding a 2-second pause in the down position; or elevating your feet further. So in Workout 2, you'll either pause 2 seconds on each rep, or raise your feet above wherever they were in Workout 1. In Workout 3, you'll either pause 4 seconds per rep, or do all your reps with your feet higher than they were in Workout 2. The exception is Workout 5. Do as many reps as possible of the original push-up variation, with no pause.

Workout B

For all exercises, use the same weight in workouts 2 and 5, but do 2 more reps per set in Workout 5 (10 instead of 8). For the incline reverse crunch, adjust the angle so it's progressively harder.

Exercise		Sets	Reps	Rest (seconds)
Alternating sets				
A1	Reverse lunge, one dumbbell on shoulder (page 178)			
	Workout 1	2	10	60
	Workout 2	3	8	60
	Workout 3	3	6	60
	Workout 4	4	4	60
	Workout 5	2	10	60
A2	Dumbbell two-point row (page 206)			
	Workout 1	2	10	60
	Workout 2	3	8	60
	Workout 3	3	6	60
	Workout 4	4	4	60
	Workout 5	2	10	60
A3	Dumbbell push press (page 186)			
	Workout 1	2	10	60
	Workout 2	3	8	60
	Workout 3	3	6	60
	Workout 4	4	4	60
	Workout 5	2	10	60
Alternating sets				
C1	Back extension (page 227)			
	Workout 1	2	10	60
	Workout 2	2	8	60
	Workout 3	3	6	60
	Workout 4	3	4	60
	Workout 5	2	10	60
C2	Incline reverse crunch (page 217)			
	Workout 1	2	10	60
	Workout 2	2	8	60
	Workout 3	3	6	60
	Workout 4	3	4	60
	Workout 5	2	10	60

Stage 7. The Final Cut

Now, for the final workouts, you'll see more big changes in the workout design. The first change is in nomenclature. Instead of calling the workouts A and B, we number them from 1 to 6. That's because you'll open the workout with either squats, a super-set of bench presses and rows, or deadlifts. But once you're past the opening exercise or exercises, you'll rotate just two different sets of exercises.

Confused?

Don't be; the workouts are laid out in the next few pages. You can do workouts 1 through 6 once each, or repeat the sequence for a total of twelve workouts. And if you get through twelve workouts in this stage, all I can say is this: You're a better man than I.

Workout 1				
Exercise		**Sets**	**Reps**	**Rest (seconds)**
A	Barbell squat (page 158)	2	6–8	90
Alternating sets				
B1	Static lunge, rear foot elevated (page 175)	4	15–20	30
B2	Push-up (page 191)	4	15–20	30
B3	Barbell Romanian deadlift (page 168)	4	15–20	30
B4	Dumbbell bent-over row (page 204)	4	15–20	30

Workout 2				
Exercise		**Sets**	**Reps**	**Rest (seconds)**
Alternating sets				
A1	Barbell incline bench press (page 193)	2	6–8	90
A2	Seated row (page 202)	2	6–8	90
Alternating sets				
B1	Dumbbell squat, heels raised on plates (page 163)	4	15–20	30
B2	Dumbbell shoulder press (page 184)	4	15–20	30
B3	Step-up (page 171)	4	15–20	30
B4	Underhand-grip lat pulldown (page 200)	4	15–20	30

Workout 3

Exercise		Sets	Reps	Rest (seconds)
A	Barbell deadlift (page 164)	2	6–8	90
Alternating sets				
B1	Static lunge, rear foot elevated (page 175)	4	15–20	30
B2	Push-up (page 191)	4	15–20	30
B3	Barbell Romanian deadlift (page 168)	4	15–20	30
B4	Dumbbell bent-over row (page 204)	4	15–20	30

Workout 4

Exercise		Sets	Reps	Rest (seconds)
A	Barbell squat (page 158)	2	6–8	90
Alternating sets				
B1	Dumbbell squat, heels raised on plates (page 163)	4	15–20	30
B2	Dumbbell shoulder press (page 185)	4	15–20	30
B3	Step-up (page 171)	4	15–20	30
B4	Underhand-grip lat pulldown (page 200)	4	15–20	30

Workout 5

Exercise		Sets	Reps	Rest (seconds)
Alternating sets				
A1	Barbell incline bench press (page 193)	2	6–8	90
A2	Seated row (page 202)	2	6–8	90
Alternating sets				
B1	Static lunge, rear foot elevated (page 175)	4	15–20	30
B2	Push-up (page 191)	4	15–20	30
B3	Barbell Romanian deadlift (page 168)	4	15–20	30
B4	Dumbbell bent-over row (page 204)	4	15–20	30

Workout 6

	Exercise	Sets	Reps	Rest (seconds)
A	Barbell deadlift (page 164)	2	6–8	90
Alternating sets				
B1	Dumbbell squat, heels raised on plates (page 163)	4	15–20	30
B2	Dumbbell shoulder press (page 185)	4	15–20	30
B3	Step-up (page 171)	4	15–20	30
B4	Underhand-grip lat pulldown (page 200)	4	15–20	30

The Right Moves

SQUAT

WHAT IT IS A fundamental human movement that mimics athletic actions like jumping, as well as everyday tasks like getting up from a chair.

WHAT MUSCLES IT WORKS Your body has more than six hundred muscles, and the squat is thought to work close to half of them. The biggest muscles in your lower body—all the lower-body muscles, really—get involved in moving your joints or stabilizing them. The biggest joint movers are the quadriceps (which straighten your knees after they're bent), hamstrings, and gluteals (which combine to straighten your hips as you rise from the bottom of the squat). There's also some movement in the ankle joint, which involves your calves, and a fierce effort by the muscles of your inner and outer thighs to keep your knees from moving in or out.

All the muscles in the middle of your body get involved to protect your spine. If you're using a barbell, holding it in front of your shoulders or behind them, you're involving muscles in your upper back, shoulders, and neck. And if you're using dumbbells, you'll get muscles in your arms and hands into the exercise.

Barbell squat (aka back squat)

GET READY: If you're not familiar with the squat rack, it's time to stop being strangers.

- Set the barbell in the rack just below the level of your shoulders.
- Grab the bar with your hands just beyond shoulder-width apart.
- Duck under the bar, pull your shoulder blades together, and rest the bar on the small shelf created by the muscles between your shoulder blades.
- Set your feet directly under the bar, about shoulder-width apart. Your knees should be slightly bent.
- Straighten your knees as you lift the bar off the supports.
- Take one step back from the supports with each foot, and set your feet shoulder-width apart, toes pointed forward.

DESCEND

- Push your hips back as if sitting in a chair, and lower yourself until your upper thighs are parallel to the floor or your lower back starts to lose its natural arch, whichever comes first.

LIFT

- Push down through the middle of your feet (not your toes), then stand straight up.

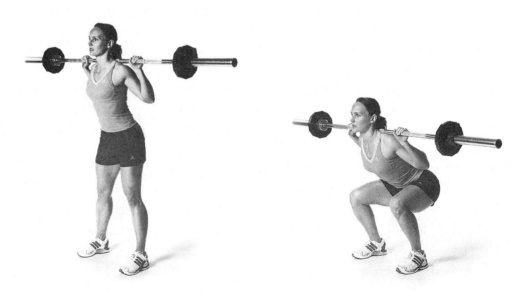

The myth of perfect form

In the winter of 2007, I chatted with a newspaper reporter who was looking into some of the arguments trainers and strength coaches conduct among themselves. We shared some of the strangest ideas we've heard about exercise form, and then he told me something he'd heard from women he knew in the media who were dedicated lifters and fitness buffs. They were all sick of the "form Nazis," the people who insist there is one way and *only* one way to do every exercise. If you deviate one degree from the prescribed angles, you deserve whatever injuries the exercise gods inflict upon your apostate muscles and connective tissues.

The problem here, as I mentioned in Chapter 1, is that different bodies have different shapes and bone lengths, as well as slight variations in range of motion due to genetic or acquired flexibility issues. If you have less flexibility in your ankle joints, for example, your squat will look a bit different from mine—you won't be able to sit back on your haunches in the bottom position, with your weight distributed evenly on your feet. You'll start to come up on your toes, which isn't what you want to do with a barbell on your shoulders. (There is a squat variation, described on page 163, in which you deliberately lift your heels off the floor while holding dumbbells. But that's a different exercise, with a different goal.) You have to stop the descent when your weight shifts to your toes, which means your range of motion will be slightly shorter than mine.

It's probably more useful to think of "ideal form," rather than perfection. Ideally, if you were to look at yourself from the side when you're in the bottom position of the squat, you'd see that your shoulder is directly over the middle of your foot. Your lower legs and torso would be at roughly the same angle in relation to the floor. That angle, however, will change from person to person. Someone with a relatively long torso and short legs would probably have more forward lean in the bottom position, with her knees out over her toes. Someone with longer legs would probably be more upright, with her knees behind her toes.

Both would be good form for that particular woman, but neither would be using "perfect" form.

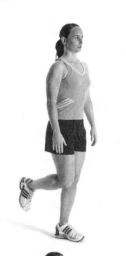

Partial single-leg squat

GET READY

- Stand with your feet hip-width apart.
- Lift your right foot off the floor behind you (or your left, if you're right-handed or your left is naturally your stronger side).
- Keep your thighs even with each other; just bend your right knee enough to get the foot off the floor.
- You can have your arms out in front of your body or to the sides, whichever is best for your balance.

DESCEND

- Push your hips back, as if you were sitting back into a chair, and lower yourself as far as you can without feeling strain in your back or knee. (Remember, it's a *partial* squat.)

LIFT

- Rise back to the starting position.
- Finish all your reps, then switch sides and repeat the set.

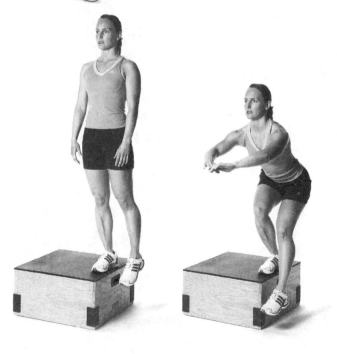

Alternative

You can do the same exercise standing on the edge of a sturdy bench or step. (I'm serious about the sturdy part.) Stand on one foot, with the other foot just off the edge. Don't bend the knee of your nonworking leg. Now, as you lower yourself, your nonworking foot will go straight down toward the floor. Some people (me, for example) find it easier to do the exercise this way, getting a better range of motion. It's up to you.

Loading up

You do the single-leg squat in phases 3 and 5, and in both programs you use fairly low reps: 6 per set in Phase 3, 4 in Phase 5. Chances are, doing these with just your body weight will be too easy, so you'll need to make them harder by holding light dumb-bells in your hands, or holding a weight plate across your chest. If you choose to add weight, make sure you do a practice set with each leg, using no additional weight.

She's a pistol!

I used to work with a woman who had been an elite figure skater. She could do single-leg squats all day with beautiful form. Moreover, she could do them with her non-working leg *straight out in front of her torso,* a variation called the "pistol squat." In the full-range-of-motion pistol squat, the thigh of the working leg touches the calf on that side. I've never been able to come close to this position, but if you've ever been a dancer, skater, gymnast, or martial artist, you might be able to. If you can do pistols with no discomfort in your back or knees, feel free to substitute them for the partial single-leg squat.

Unilateral maneuvers

When doing an exercise that works one leg or arm at a time, always start with your nondominant side. So if you're right-handed, that's your dominant side, and you should start out with your left leg or arm. If you've had an injury to your dominant side, and it's now weaker than your nondominant limb, then start with the weaker one. Your goal is to match the repetitions you do with the weaker or nondominant limb with your stronger or dominant side. If you did it the other way around, you might do more reps per set with your stronger side, and exacerbate the imbalance.

Dumbbell single-arm overhead squat

GET READY

- Get two dumbbells, one twice as heavy as the other. So if one is 5 pounds, the other is 10 pounds.
- Stand with your feet shoulder-width apart and toes pointed straight ahead.
- Hold the light dumbbell overhead (actually, slightly behind your head) in your nondominant hand, with the heavier dumbbell between your legs at arm's length.

DESCEND

- Push your hips back and lower yourself until your upper thighs are parallel to the floor, holding the lighter dumbbell straight up over your shoulders.

LIFT

- Rise back to the start position.
- Do all your reps, then switch arms and repeat the set.

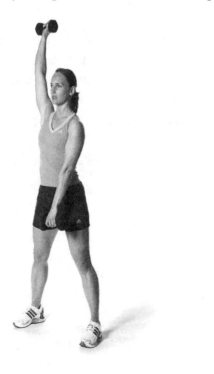
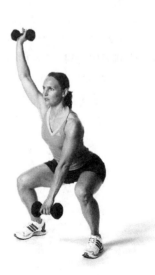

Dumbbell squat, heels raised on plates

GET READY

- Set two weight plates on the floor (10-pound plates should work well) so you can stand on them with your feet shoulder-width apart.
- Grab two dumbbells, and hold them at your sides at arm's length as you stand with your heels on the plates.

DESCEND

- Push your hips back and lower yourself until your upper thighs are parallel to the floor.

LIFT

- Rise back to the starting position.

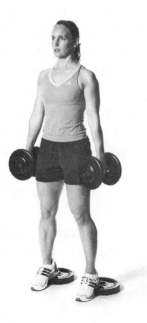 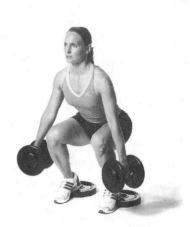

Plate tectonics

Why the plates under the heels? In theory, doing squats with heels elevated shifts more of the work to the vastus medialis, one of the four quadriceps muscles, which has a role in protecting your knees.

If you're up for a challenge, try doing the exercise on your toes, without the plates under your heels. That's a variation Alwyn learned from the late Mel Siff, Ph.D. You probably want to do it without weights, at least at first.

DEADLIFT

WHAT IT IS Another fundamental human movement, the deadlift is perhaps the most useful gym exercise in existence. It mimics the action of picking up something heavy off the floor, which is pretty much your entire life if you're the mother of young children. Even if you're not, you're still a woman, which means the muscles on the back of your body are probably weaker than they should be, relative to the muscles on the front. The deadlift and its variations, more than any other exercises, correct that imbalance.

WHAT MUSCLES IT WORKS The primary action is called "hip extension"—straightening your hips when your torso is bent forward. It shares that action with the squat, which means it works many of the same muscles, especially the hamstrings and gluteals. But the muscles of the upper and middle back get more directly involved. The diamond-shaped trapezius—which runs from the base of your skull, out to your shoulder blades, and down to the middle of your back—is responsible for pulling your shoulder blades together (among other tasks, explained later in this chapter). With a heavy load in your hands, pulling your arms down and your shoulder blades farther apart, you can see how hard those muscles have to work to pull your shoulders back.

Naturally, everything in the middle of your body that works hard in a squat works at least as hard in a deadlift. You must maintain the natural arch in your lower back, and the heavier the weight you lift off the floor, the harder it is for those muscles to protect your spine. (Remember, "harder" is better when it comes to improving your body in appearance and function.)

You also work the gripping muscles in your hands and forearms. Remember back in Chapter 2, when I said that grip strength was correlated with longevity—that is, *not dying*? Well, here's the best way to strengthen that grip.

Barbell deadlift

GET READY

- Load an Olympic barbell (the 45-pound, 7-foot-long bar) and set it on the floor.
- Stand with the bar against your shins, your feet about shoulder-width apart and your toes pointed forward.

- Squat down and grab it with an overhand grip, your hands just outside your legs.
- Straighten your arms and tighten everything, from your shoulders to your feet. Don't be afraid to grab the bar like you're mad at it.
- Look straight ahead, rather than down at the bar or up at the ceiling.

LIFT

- Pull the bar straight up your shins as you stand.
- Once the bar is past your knees, push your hips forward and pull your shoulder blades together in back.
- Pause in this top position.

DESCEND

- Slide the weight back down your legs to the floor. You'll want to control the speed to avoid a sudden jolt to your lower-back muscles. But you don't have to lower the bar at any particular speed—just get it down to the floor. (If you've ever been in a gym with elite strength athletes, you know they simply drop the weight when they've completed a repetition with a near-maximum weight. Unfortunately, idiots sometimes do this as well, without any good reason beyond the fact that they're idiots.)
- On your heaviest sets, let the bar come to a complete stop on the floor, and reset your grip and posture before lifting again. On higher-rep sets, let the weights tap the floor before beginning the next repetition.

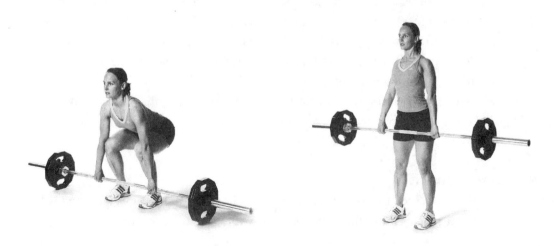

Strapped? Or strapless?

If you've spent a lot of time in gyms, you've probably seen lifting straps. These are bands designed to help you hold onto a bar that you might otherwise drop due to limits in the strength or endurance of your gripping muscles. They're usually made from canvas, leather, or a nylon-acrylic blend, and are sometimes tricked out with neoprene or some other padding.

Bodybuilders tend to use them for every exercise that involves a pulling motion—deadlifts, chin-ups, rows, shrugs. I used to use them, but abandoned the straps (along with my lifting belt) when I realized that it made more sense to develop enough strength to lift heavy things without straps and belts. After a few months, I could lift more without those props than I could with them.

You, though, might benefit from using straps from time to time, especially if you notice that your grip strength gives out on you before the muscles in your back or hips feel as if they've been fully challenged.

A quick online scan showed that prices range from six to thirty dollars with more options in length, width, and padding than I ever knew existed. If you don't want to risk the vagaries of the Internet, you can probably find a set at a local sporting-goods store that sells strength-training equipment. Harbinger and Schiek are the most popular brands.

Wide-grip deadlift from box

GET READY

- Load a barbell and set it on the floor in front of a low box or step. (You want it to be about three to four inches above the floor.)
- Stand on the box, your feet shoulder-width apart, toes pointed forward. Squat down and roll the barbell up to your toes. Grab the bar overhand with a wide grip, about double shoulder width.
- Tighten up your body and your grip. You want to be in the position I described earlier for the barbell deadlift, only with knees bent more and hips closer to the floor.

ALTERNATIVE SETUP

- If you can't roll the bar up over your toes—if you have smaller weights on the bar, so the bar sits lower than the step—then you need to get off the box, roll the bar forward, squat down and pick it up with the wide grip, and then step back up onto the box. Set your feet the way I described.

- Squat down as described below under "Descend," and then begin the first repetition.

LIFT

- Pull the bar straight up your shins as you stand.
- Once the bar is past your knees, push your hips forward and pull your shoulder blades together in back.
- Pause in this top position.

DESCEND

- Lower the bar until the bottom edges of the weight plates are just below the level of the step or box. In other words, don't lower it all the way to the floor on every repetition. You want just a little more range of motion than you get with conventional deadlifts.

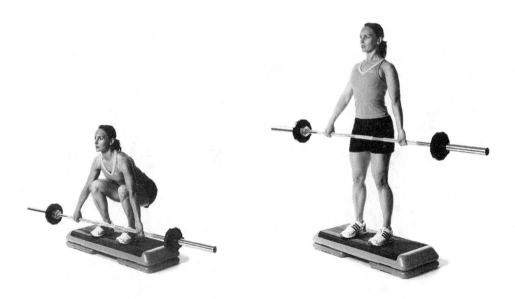

Barbell Romanian deadlift

GET READY

- Load a barbell and set it on the floor.
- Stand over the bar with your feet shoulder-width apart, and grab it with an overhand, shoulder-width grip.
- Lift it as you would a deadlift, and stand with the bar at arm's length against your front thighs.

DESCEND

- Lower the bar along your thighs until it's just below your knees.
- Keep your back in its natural arch by pushing your hips back and allowing your knees to bend a bit.

LIFT

- Push your hips forward as you straighten your torso and pull the bar back to the starting position.

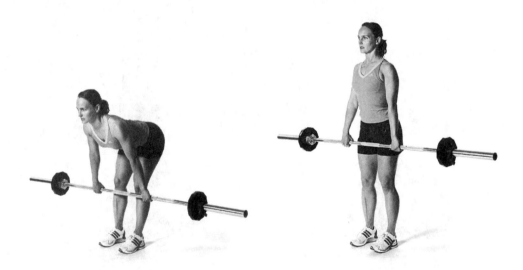

Commie cred

You may wonder why this exercise is a "Romanian" deadlift, as opposed to, say, a "partial" deadlift, or something more descriptive of the exercise itself. The short answer is that it was actually invented by Romanian Olympic weight lifters and their coaches as a back-strengthening exercise. (Because of the shorter range of motion, there's more direct involvement of the muscles in the lower back, gluteals, and hamstrings than in a conventional deadlift, and less work for the trapezius.) I learned that from Terry Todd, Ph.D., a historian at the University of Texas and former world-class power lifter.

The long answer is that, for many years, American lifters and coaches were so convinced that their Eastern Bloc counterparts were so far ahead in training methodology that they'd jump at anything that had the imprimatur of the Big Red sports machine.

Other exercises you see in this program have more dubious claims to their Marxist monikers. Todd told me there's no evidence that the Bulgarian split squat (page 176) came from Bulgaria. But he added that there is such a thing as a Bulgarian step-up—it's similar to the step-up shown on page 171, but the step is higher and you'd use a barbell instead of dumbbells. And it was battle-tested by actual Bulgarians (on the advice of a Russian trainer), who found it superior to the squat for helping them build strength and muscle mass.

The Cuban press also has Russian origins—it was used in Cuba, but only after Russian coaches taught them the exercise. (Alwyn's version, shown on page 207, is a variation on the original exercise, which is performed standing up and using a barbell.)

Curiously, a well-known abdominal exercise called the Russian twist (not included in these programs) actually has Western roots. British soldiers were using a version of it as far back as the nineteenth century, according to Todd.

Dumbbell single-leg Romanian deadlift

GET READY
- Grab a pair of light dumbbells and hold them at your sides as you stand with your feet hip-width apart.

DESCEND
- Bend forward at the hips as you extend one leg behind you.
- Lower the weights until they're just past the knee of your working leg.
- Your body should form a straight line from the heel of the leg that's extended behind you to your neck, with your arms hanging straight down from your shoulders, and parallel to your working leg.

LIFT
- Return to the starting position.
- Do all the repetitions with the same working leg (your weaker or nondominant leg) and then switch sides and repeat the set.

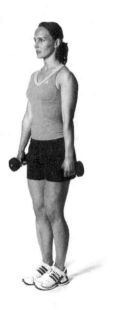
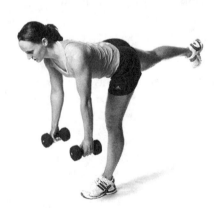

STEP-UP AND LUNGE

WHAT THEY ARE In the gym, most exercises that focus on your lower body are done with your feet parallel to each other. Whether you're doing squats or deadlifts or (like so many tragically unenlightened lifters) leg presses, extensions, and curls, the feet are usually next-door neighbors, and your legs are moving in tandem.

But in real life, few actions involve such a convenient placement of your feet. After all, you don't hop on two feet to get from one place to the next. Walking, running, and climbing require your feet to be on different lines, if not different planes. Virtually every sport calls for lunging actions—forward, back, sideways, and every angle in between.

If that's the way you move in real life, it makes sense to work your muscles in those directions in the gym. And, in truth, it's not hard to get women to do these exercises. (Guys? Well, that's a different story.) Still, Alwyn goes farther than most in working these actions from a variety of angles and planes, as you noticed in the squat and deadlift sections. You'll like the aesthetic results, since these unique exercises hit your lower-body muscles from directions you didn't know existed. And if you notice that the everyday things you do suddenly seem easier, that's even better.

WHAT MUSCLES THEY WORK Everything in your lower body gets worked in lunges and step-ups. And in keeping with Alwyn's program-design philosophy, every exercise that develops coordination and balance is also a "core" exercise, meaning your midbody muscles have to work to keep your back and pelvis properly aligned.

Step-up

GET READY

- Grab a pair of dumbbells and a step or bench. The higher the step, the harder the exercise will be.
- Stand in front of the step with your feet hip-width apart, holding the dumbbells at your sides.
- Place the foot of your nondominant leg on the step, with your foot flat.

LIFT

- Push down through the heel of the foot on the step and lift yourself up so your trailing leg is even with your working leg.

- Brush the step with your nonworking foot. (In other words, don't rest your weight on that foot on the step; keep all your weight on your working leg.)

DESCEND
- Lower your nonworking leg to the starting position.
- Finish the set, then switch legs and repeat.

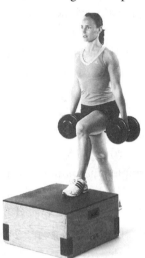
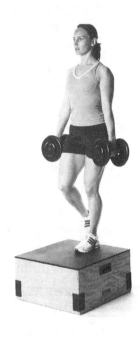

Leg work

Remember that your trailing leg is just along for the ride. You want the working leg to do all the work. (Which is why we call it the "working" leg, in case you didn't guess that already.) Consciously push down through the foot on the step on each repetition so you avoid the temptation to use your trailing leg for assistance.

Extra credit

You can make the exercise harder by using a barbell instead of dumbbells. Hold it across your shoulders as you would in a barbell squat. The set-up is a little trickier with a barbell. What I do is set the bar on uprights in a rack, just as I would for a squat, but I approach it with my back, instead of facing it and ducking my head under the bar to get started. I set the step in front of the squat rack, so after I unrack the bar, I only need to take one or two short strides to reach the step. The exercise works the same way from that point, although I'll note that you have to be more careful as you step down. The bar on your back changes your center of gravity, so your body descends faster than you expect or want it to, and the more tired you get, the harder it is to control that descent.

That said, it's an incredible exercise for leg-muscle development. And it does wonders for improving your focus in the gym. If you space out with a barbell on your shoulders and one foot off the floor . . . well, let's just say concentration is even more important than usual on a barbell step-up.

Lunge

GET READY

- Grab a pair of dumbbells and hold them at your sides as you stand with your feet hip-width apart.

DESCEND

- Take a long step forward with your nondominant leg, and lower your body until the upper thigh of that leg is parallel to the floor.
- The knee of your trailing leg should almost touch the floor.
- Your torso remains upright, with your shoulders square and your eyes forward.

LIFT

- Push back to the starting position.
- Repeat with your opposite leg forward, and continue to alternate until you've done all the repetitions with each leg.

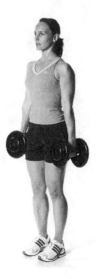
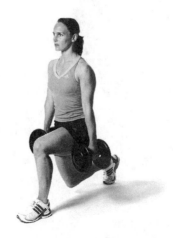

Barbell split squat

GET READY

- Set up a barbell in the squat rack and position it on your shoulders, as described previously for the barbell squat (page 158).
- Step back from the rack, and then take one long step forward or backward, as if you were going to do a lunge.

DESCEND

- Lower yourself until the upper thigh of your front leg is perpendicular to the floor, and the knee of your trailing leg nearly touches the floor.
- Keep your torso upright, with your midbody muscles tight and shoulders pulled back.

LIFT

- Push back up to the starting, split-leg position.
- Do all your reps, then repeat the set with the other leg forward.

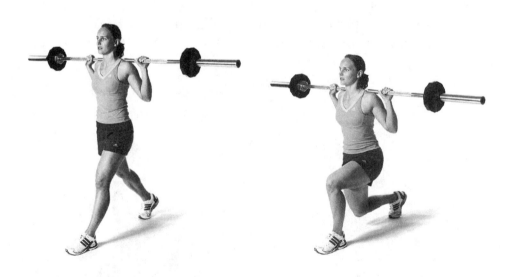

Static lunge, rear foot elevated

GET READY

- Grab a pair of dumbbells and a low step.
- Set the toes of your dominant leg on the step, as if they were on the starting block at a track meet.
- Take a long stride forward with your nondominant leg.
- Hold the dumbbells at your sides, with your torso upright and eyes forward.

DESCEND

- Lower yourself until the top of the thigh of your forward leg is parallel to the floor.
- Push back up to the starting position.
- Finish all your repetitions, then repeat the set with your opposite leg.

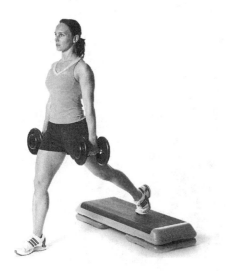
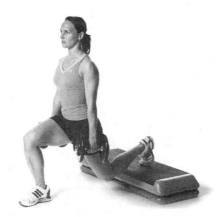

Bulgarian split squat

GET READY

- Grab a weight plate, medicine ball, or dumbbell and stand in front of a bench.
- Set the top of your dominant foot on the bench.
- Take a stride forward with your nondominant leg.
- Hold the weight against your chest, with your torso upright, shoulders square, and eyes forward.

DESCEND

- Lower yourself until the upper thigh of your forward leg is parallel to the floor.

LIFT

- Push back up to the starting position.
- Finish all your repetitions, then repeat the set with your opposite leg.

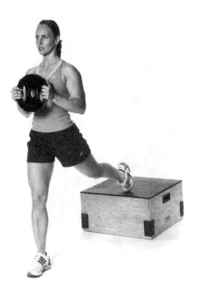 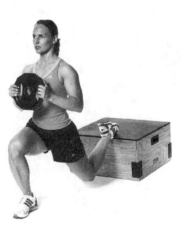

Reverse lunge from box with forward reach

GET READY

- Grab a pair of light dumbbells and a low step or box.
- Stand on the box, holding the dumbbells at your sides.

DESCEND

- Step back with your dominant leg and reach toward the toes of your front foot with the dumbbells.
- Your front thigh should be parallel to the floor as the dumbbells reach your front foot.

LIFT

- Push back to the starting position.
- Finish all your repetitions, then repeat the set with your opposite leg.

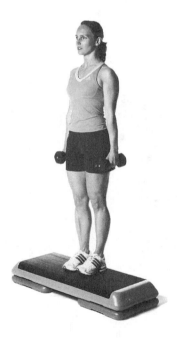
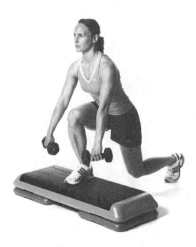

Reverse lunge, one dumbbell on shoulder

GET READY

- Grab a dumbbell and hold it at your left shoulder, as if you were going to do a shoulder press with it. That is, you want your palm facing out, and the inside edge of the dumbbell should be just above the outside edge of your shoulder.
- Stand with your feet hip-width apart.

DESCEND

- Step back with your right leg, and lower your body until your left thigh is parallel to the floor and your right knee nearly touches the floor.

LIFT

- Push back up to the starting position.
- Finish all the reps, then repeat the set with the dumbbell at your right shoulder, stepping back with your left leg.

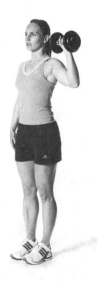 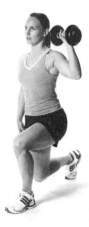

Offsetting gains

Working with an unbalanced load—making your body heavier on one side than the other—is one of the oddest-looking but most effective ways to improve core strength. As Alwyn explains, you can easily walk across the room while carrying two equal-size weights. But try walking across the room carrying a single weight that's as heavy as the two equal-size weights combined. You're carrying the same load, but if the weight is unbalanced, it's much harder to use. That means your body will have to get stronger to compensate.

This isn't a technique you want to use if you're just starting out, which is why it appears in Stage 6. By that point, you'll be ready for a challenge that goes beyond the normal-looking exercises.

COMBINATION UPPER-BODY/LOWER-BODY EXERCISES

WHAT THEY ARE Most human movements involve a combination of upper- and lower-body actions. But in the gym, we have a bias toward bisection—treating our bodies as if they could function perfectly well if we sawed them in half somewhere between the ribs and pelvis.

The exercises in the previous sections involve your upper body as a supporting player, usually as a kind of scaffold for whatever weights you're using to build lower-body muscles.

The two exercises in this section make you move the weights with coordinated action of your northern and southern hemispheres. Of course that involves more muscle mass, which means it burns more calories. But it also helps you develop balance and coordination, which translate into more overall strength, power, and physical grace. If you've ever admired the way an athlete moves, you know what I mean.

WHICH MUSCLES THEY USE The muscles involved in an overhead press and snatch are described in the next section. And the lower-body muscles used in these two exercises are the ones described earlier—pretty much all of them, in other words.

The difference with these two exercises is the *way* you use the same muscles. Whereas the exercises in the rest of this chapter are meant to be done at a deliberate pace—usually 3 to 4 seconds per repetition—these are meant to be done with fast, explosive actions. Your goal is to develop muscle power, which is related to muscle strength but has a slightly different context.

Strength is the ability to exert force—to move something heavy, regardless of the speed at which it's moved. Power is the ability to move something as fast as possible, and it matters more than most of us realize. As you get older it declines faster than strength or muscle mass. Some of the really smart people I've spoken to over the years think that the loss of power has the biggest impact on our quality of life as we get older.

It's impossible to separate strength and power entirely—the strongest people tend to be able to generate the most power. For that matter, muscle mass and strength are generally correlated, as well. But there's something about the ability to generate power that sets it apart—the faster we lose that ability, the faster we get old and frail. That's why the most forward-thinking coaches, like Alwyn, include power-generating exercises like push presses and snatches in their training programs, even if the trainee has no ambitions to run faster, jump higher, or throw a ball harder.

We're all going to get old, if we're lucky enough to live that long. And we're all going to die. But if it's within our power to make those things happen later, instead of sooner, why not use exercises like these to put the brakes on the aging process?

Front squat/push press

GET READY

- Set up a barbell on the uprights in a squat rack. You want it lower than your setting for the back squat, probably at about your midchest.
- Grab the barbell with an overhand grip that's just beyond shoulder width.
- As you lift it off the rack, lift your elbows straight up in front of your torso; your upper arms and torso should form a 90-degree angle at the shoulders, with your upper arms perpendicular to your torso. This sets the barbell in a natural groove formed by the front parts of your deltoid muscles.
- Allow the bar to roll from your palms to your fingers. It seems awkward at first, but it's the best way to hold the bar in the proper position.
- Step back as you would for a typical barbell squat, with your feet shoulder-width apart, toes pointed forward, and eyes focused straight ahead.

DESCEND

- Lower yourself until your upper thighs are parallel to the floor.
- Keep your torso as upright as possible. (I don't really need to remind you of this. The slightest forward lean throws off your balance, which becomes immediately apparent the first time you try the exercise. Your body will catch on fast.)

LIFT

- Push back up to the starting position.
- As you get near the top, before your knees are straight, start to press the barbell straight up overhead, moving your head back just enough for the bar to get past it. Unlike a regular shoulder press, you want to use your momentum from the squat to get the bar moving up off your shoulders.
- To do the press, you'll need to lower your elbows, which will allow the bar to roll back down to your palms.
- Straighten your knees, and use your upward momentum to rise up onto your toes. It's as if you were trying to throw the weight up through the ceiling, although you'd be insane to let go of the bar at this point.
- Pause with your arms fully extended overhead, then lower the bar to your shoulders and immediately descend for the next repetition.

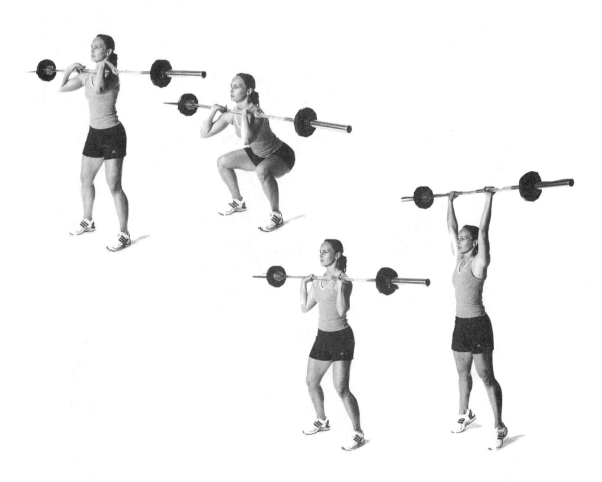

Barbell Romanian deadlift/bent-over row

GET READY

- Load a barbell and set it on the floor.
- Stand over the bar with your feet shoulder-width apart, and grab it with an overhand, shoulder-width grip.
- Lift as you would a deadlift, and stand with the bar at arm's length against your front thighs.

DESCEND

- Lower the bar along your thighs until it's just below your knees.
- Keep your back in its natural arch by pushing your hips back and allowing your knees to bend a bit.

LIFT

- Pull the bar to your upper abdomen, keeping your torso and lower body in the same positions.
- Slowly lower the bar until it's just below your knees again.
- Push your hips forward as you straighten your torso and pull the bar back to the front of your thighs.
- That's one repetition. Repeat by lowering the bar as you push your hips back and bend your knees.

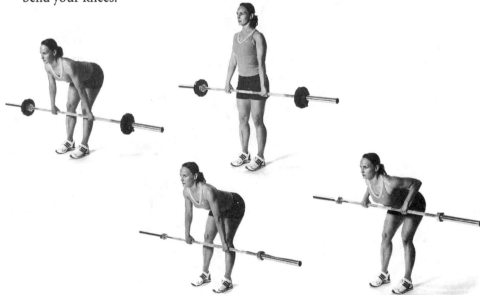

One-armed dumbbell snatch

GET STARTED

- Grab a dumbbell with your nondominant hand, and make sure you have a little elbow room. You don't want to be crowded when you're moving a weight at full speed.
- Set your feet shoulder-width apart, toes pointed forward.
- Squat down, holding the dumbbell between your legs with a straight arm. (Your nondominant hand can do whatever feels natural to improve your balance.)

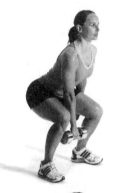

LIFT

- Jump, or at least push yourself up so fast you come all the way up on your toes.
- Keep your arm loose, and let the force generated by your jump get the dumbbell moving up the front of your torso.
- Steer the dumbbell until it's straight up over your head. Don't think about the muscles you're using to make this happen. As with the push press, it's as if you were throwing the weight overhead, without actually letting go. (*Please* don't let go of the weight.)

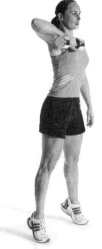

DESCEND

- Once your arm is fully extended overhead, hold for a second to make sure your body is stable. Then lower the dumbbell, and drop down into the starting position.
- Do all your reps with your nondominant arm, then repeat with your other arm.

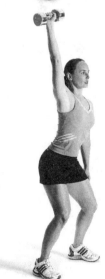

PRESSING EXERCISES

WHAT THEY ARE If you push a weight away from your body, it falls into one of three broad categories:

- Chest presses, in which you push the weight away from your body at an angle perpendicular to your torso.
- Dips, in which you push down to move your body up. (This exercise can be tough on your shoulders, which is one reason why Alwyn doesn't include it in these programs.)
- Shoulder presses, in which you push a weight straight up from your shoulders.

WHAT MUSCLES THEY WORK In truth, all presses are "shoulder" presses, in that most of the muscles involved act on the major joints of the shoulder complex. We call the overhead press a "shoulder" press because it has the most direct effect on your deltoids, the muscles that cover your ball-and-socket shoulder joint. When you lift your arms up and away from your torso, the deltoids are the most obvious muscles involved.

A chest press works your pectoral muscles, although the front part of the deltoid helps pull your arms up and out over your torso.

You complete these movements by straightening your elbows, an action provided by your triceps.

The final bit of muscular magic involves your shoulder blades, which are pulled out away from each other on a chest press, and rotate out and up on an overhead press. The actions of the shoulder blades—the scapulae, if you don't mind some gratuitous Latin—are important to everything we do, but they get hardly any attention at all. They float freely over the back of your rib cage, pulled up, down, together, and apart by some of your body's strongest muscles. The trapezius, which I described in the "Deadlift" section, is the main one, but there are many more, with names that sound like a mix of Gregorian chant and *Jurassic Park*. (Seriously, I bet that if a trainer told his client that a new exercise would work his *Dominus vobiscum,* with support from his *Tyrannosaurus minor,* he could pull it off.)

Speaking of the shoulder blades, here's one of my pet peeves:

When you approach the dumbbell rack of any gym in America, you see a bunch of people doing a bunch of lifts with their backs fully supported by exercise benches—a technique that hinders the movement of the shoulder blades. I suspect a lot of the people doing back-supported shoulder presses have never once tried a shoulder press without back support, much less standing on their own two feet.

The shoulder blades are crucial to everything you do with your shoulders, which is to say everything you do with your upper body. Exercises like standing shoulder presses allow them to move freely and do their jobs. Blocking their actions, as you would in a back-supported shoulder press, forces all your working parts to move in unnatural ways to make up for the inaction of the shoulder blades.

I just can't understand why anyone thinks that's a good idea.

Dumbbell shoulder press

GET READY

- Grab a pair of dumbbells and stand with your feet shoulder-width apart.
- Hold the dumbbells with a palms-out grip, the weights at the edges of your shoulder muscles.
- You want your knees slightly bent, your lower back in its natural arch, your shoulders square.

LIFT

- Push the weights straight up from your shoulders.
- Pause at the top; make sure you feel the contraction in your triceps muscles.

DESCEND

- Lower the weights to the start-ing position.

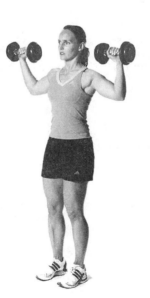
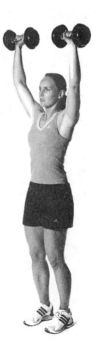

Build your muscles, save your eardrums

If you spend a lot of time in gyms, like me, you occasionally see lifters who seem to think that the more noise they make, the more muscle they build. Thus, they clank dumbbells overhead on every repetition of the dumbbell shoulder press.

Think about it: You build muscle by working against the forces of gravity. If gravity isn't providing any resistance, there's no work for your muscles to do. And the final part of the "clank press" involves no gravitational resistance whatsoever. You could hold two metal things overhead and bang them against each other for hours on end, until you either burst your eardrums or got shot by your neighbor who works third shift and sleeps during the day.

But if you lift weights straight overhead, you're working against gravity through the entire range of motion, which makes a lot more sense, for your muscles as well as your eardrums.

Dumbbell push press

GET READY

- Grab a pair of dumbbells and stand holding them at your shoulders, as described above.

DESCEND

- Bend at the knees and hips, as if you were about to jump.

LIFT

- As you snap your hips forward and straighten your knees, use that momentum to push the weights up off your shoulders. You should come all the way up onto your toes.

DESCEND

- Lower the weights to your shoulders.

Alternative

You can do this exercise with a barbell, if you prefer. The action is the same one I described for the second half of the front squat/push press on page 180.

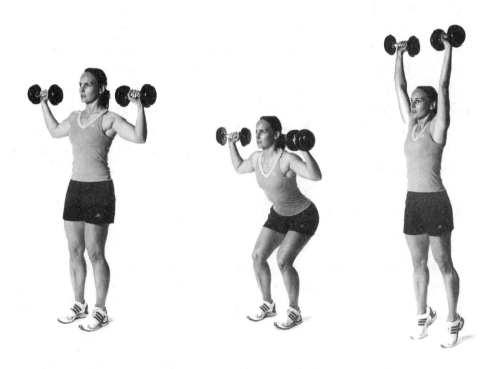

Fully loaded

This is a combined strength-and-power exercise, which means you want to use a bit more weight than you'd be able to lift on a standard shoulder press. You also want to move the weights faster. They may not actually move faster, especially as they get near the top of the lift, but the key is to try.

PUSH-UP VARIATIONS

This exercise is unique among the presses, in that we include five different versions, and invite you to choose the one that's most appropriate for the required repetitions. They're listed here from easiest to hardest, and your goals are pretty simple. First, use harder variations when the workout calls for lower reps, and easier variations for higher reps. Second, try to move up to harder variations from workout to workout, so if you start off doing the 45-degree push-up when the workout calls for 10 reps, try to advance to the 30-degree push-up in subsequent 10-rep workouts.

You'll notice that we don't use the push-up from the knees, the traditional variation pawned off on the "weaker" sex. Alwyn doesn't like it because it takes the core out of the movement. Your midbody muscles get a break when you cut yourself off at the knees. When your weight is resting on your toes and hands, and everything else is in play, your core muscles have to do the work they're designed to do.

60-degree push-up (not shown)

GET READY

- Find a counter or similarly sturdy surface that allows you to form a 60-degree angle (more or less) when your chest is at the edge of it and your feet are perhaps thirty-six inches back. (If you're in a commercial gym, you can use the bar of a Smith machine—it's the barbell-on-rails device—for this or either of the next two variations.)
- Set your hands on the edge of the surface, with your arms straight and about shoulder-width apart.
- You want your feet back about thirty-six inches from the surface, hip-width apart.
- Your weight should be balanced on your toes and hands, with your body forming a straight line from your ankles to your neck.

DESCEND

- Lower your chest to the surface, keeping everything else in the same alignment.
- Keep your elbows in, next to your ribs, rather than allowing them to flare out away from your torso.

LIFT

- Push back up to the starting position.

45-degree push-up

GET READY

- Find a sturdy object that's about hip height, and set up on it as described above. Your feet will be back a little farther from your hands this time, due to the angle.

DESCEND

- Lower your chest to the bench, keeping the rest of your body in the same alignment. At this point, your body should be at about a 45-degree angle to the floor.
- Keep your elbows in, next to your ribs, rather than allowing them to flare out away from your torso.

LIFT

- Push back to the starting position.

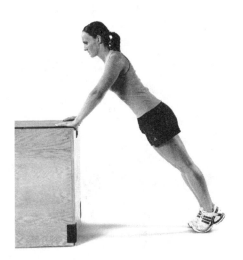
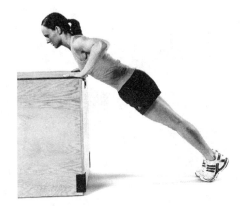

30-degree push-up

GET READY

- Find a bench or box that's sturdy and stable (it will support your weight and won't slide out from under you) and about twelve to fifteen inches high.
- Set your hands on the edge or the surface, whichever seems to offer the best support.
- Align your body as described above.

DESCEND

- Lower your chest until it's an inch or so above the surface.
- Keep your elbows in, next to your ribs, rather than allowing them to flare out away from your torso.
- Pay attention to your body alignment—the lower the angle, the more of a core exercise it becomes.

LIFT

- Push back up to the starting position.

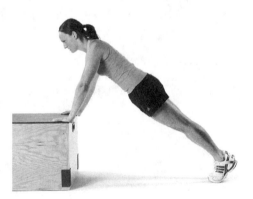 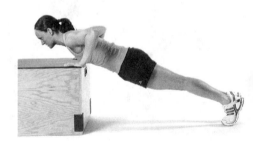

Push-up

GET READY

- Position yourself on the floor, with your weight resting on your hands and toes.
- Your hands should be about shoulder-width apart. You can move them closer or farther apart for comfort, although you change the emphasis of the exercise if you move them within a few inches of each other or significantly widen your spread. The former works your triceps harder, while the latter works your chest more (and is probably a bit tougher on your shoulder joints).
- Your body should form a straight line from your ankles to your neck. Your back should still form its natural S-curve, and of course your gluteals will rise above the line. The key is to have a line that's a straight shot from your ankles to the base of your skull, neatly bisecting your torso.

DESCEND

- Lower yourself until your chest is two to four inches from the floor (with apologies for thinking like a guy, the size of your chest will help determine your range of motion here).
- Keep your elbows in, next to your ribs, rather than allowing them to flare out away from your torso.

LIFT

- Push back up to the starting position. It's actually okay to exaggerate your range of motion at the top of the movement; it's a good workout for the serratus muscles on the sides of your rib cage.

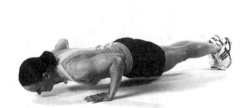
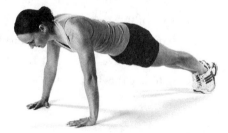

T push-up

GET READY

- Set yourself in the push-up position described above.

DESCEND

- Lower yourself to within a few inches of the floor.

LIFT

- As you push back up to the starting position, twist to your left, so your left arm ends up straight over your right, and your body and arms form a T. Your weight will all rest on your right hand and the side of your right foot (your left foot might not come all the way off the floor, but it also won't support your weight in this position).
- Let your eyes follow your left hand, so you're looking up at it in the top position.

DESCEND

- Twist back and lower your left hand to the floor, so you're back in the starting position for the classic push-up.
- Lower yourself again.

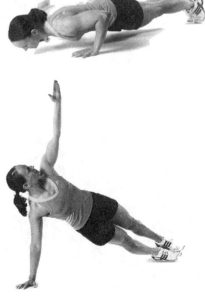

LIFT

- Twist to your right as you raise yourself, so your right arm ends up pointing toward the ceiling, and your weight is on your left hand and the outside of your left foot.
- That's two push-ups. You need to do an even number of twists to your left and right in each set, which means that if a set calls for 5 repetitions, you have to extend that to 6 if you're going to use the T push-up.

And just in case that's not hard enough . . .

You can add resistance on a T push-up by holding a dumbbell in the hand that you're raising off the floor. If you get to that level, do half your repetitions consecutively with the dumbbell in one hand, then switch and finish the set with the dumbbell in the other hand. Then again, if you're really morphing into an Amazon, you can do it with two dumbbells, and alternate on each repetition. (Just make sure the dumbbells are hexagonal, so they don't roll out from under you.)

Barbell incline bench press

GET READY

- Most gyms will have an adjustable incline bench with uprights attached to hold the barbell. Set the back of the bench to an angle that's between 30 and 45 degrees, and load the barbell.
- Lie on your back on the bench with your feet flat on the floor.
- Grab the bar with an overhand grip and your hands just beyond shoulder-width apart.
- Lift the bar off the uprights and hold it so your arms are perpendicular to the floor. The bar will probably be over your collarbones.

DESCEND

- Lower the bar to your upper chest.

LIFT

- Push the bar straight back to the starting position.

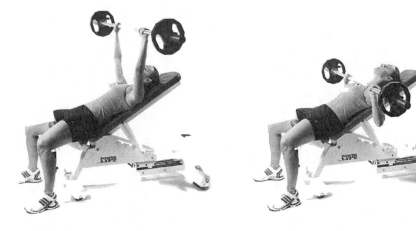

Winging it

A few pages back, I railed against the widespread use of back support on shoulder presses. So now you might ask why bench presses are any better. If anything, they block the natural actions of the shoulder blades to an even greater extent, since more of your body's weight is resting on them, along with the weight of the barbell.

The short answer is, you're right.

That's why Alwyn puts so much emphasis on the push-up, a superior exercise for two important reasons:

- It works your midbody muscles, which don't have to support any of your weight on the bench press (that's what the bench is for).
- It allows your shoulder blades to move freely.

The long answer is that you don't really use your shoulder blades in the bench press as much as you'd think. As you get stronger and more serious about lifting, you'll learn to pull your shoulder blades together in back, and hold them there throughout the lift. That technique shortens the range of motion, which in turn allows you to lift more weight.

If you do nothing but bench presses—if you never mix in push-ups and standing shoulder presses, which allow free scapular movement—you'll eventually mess up your shoulders. ("Mess up" is a technical term, denoting self-imposed physiological dysfunction.) Even worse, you could feel the injury in your neck, rather than your shoulders, and never suspect it had anything to do with too much bench pressing.

Dumbbell incline bench press

GET READY

- Set the back of an incline bench to an angle that's between 30 and 45 degrees.
- Grab a pair of dumbbells and lie on your back on the bench, with your feet flat on the floor.
- Hold the weights straight up, so your arms are perpendicular to the floor.

DESCEND

- Lower the weights to the outsides of your shoulders—that is, the inside edges of the dumbbells should be directly above the outside edges of your shoulders.
- The weights will probably stop two to four inches above your deltoids; there's no need to exaggerate the range of motion, just as there's no reason to cut it short.

LIFT

- Push the weights back up to the starting position. They'll probably be close to each other at the top, but they shouldn't touch.

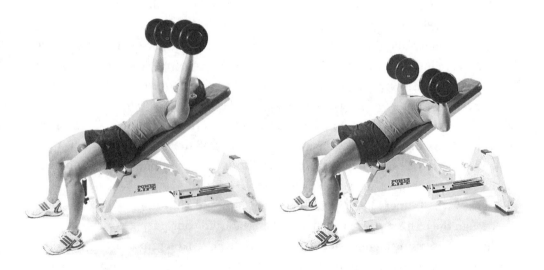

PULLING EXERCISES

WHAT THEY ARE In the broadest sense, these are the opposites of the pressing exercises already described. A lat pulldown is the reverse of a shoulder press, and a seated or bent-over row is the opposite of a push-up or bench press. Functionally, the exercises in this category are meant to mimic the actions of climbing (a vertical pull) and rowing or, say, tug-of-war (horizontal pulls).

There's also another type of exercise in this section, which could be described as "prehabilitation," or shoring up weak links before they become broken links. These exercises employ muscular actions that aren't meant to mimic anything you do in everyday life (unless your job calls on you to lie facedown on a bench and lift light weights up and down in a variety of flapping motions). Their goal is to strengthen particular muscles involved in actions like climbing and rowing.

WHAT MUSCLES THEY WORK Any entry-level bodybuilder could tell you that a lat pulldown works the lats. And most could tell you that the lats, short for latissimus dorsi, are upper-body muscles that give a bodybuilder a wider "spread" in his back. But those muscles have more than ornamental value. The thickest parts are beneath your armpits, on the sides of your torso, so of course that's what bodybuilders focus on. The thin parts include the diagonal connective tissues that run all the way to your lower back. Thus, the lats have an indirect but interesting role in protecting your spine.

If you watch someone doing pull-ups, you can see the mechanism in action. Her shoulders are pulled back, her lats are straining, and her lower back and gluteals are tightly flexed. The lower back and gluteals aren't the prime movers in the exercise, but they're clearly doing *something*. It's not going too far out on a limb to say those muscles are all doing what they'd do if you were climbing a tree or scaling a cliff. So even though you're hanging in space during a pull-up, and all the movement is being provided by the muscles in your arms and surrounding your shoulders, your middle- and lower-body muscles are still engaged.

That's why trainers like Alwyn prefer pull-ups and chin-ups to lat pulldowns. (Although the terms are often used interchangeably, for our purposes a chin-up is a pulling exercise using an underhand grip versus the overhand grip of a pull-up. Most of us are stronger on chin-ups than pull-ups.) Once you sit down on a bench and lock your knees under a pad that's in front of your torso, you're disengaging muscles that are designed to work together.

The obvious problem is that it's an extraordinarily difficult exercise for women to perform—not surprising when you consider that many men can't do a single pull-up.

The female athletes Alwyn trains can all do them (Rachel Cosgrove, Alwyn's wife, once did twelve chin-ups for an exercise DVD; Alwyn says she wasn't even out of breath), and his female clients learn to do them over time. Heck, my nine-year-old daughter taught herself to do full-range-of-motion pull-ups, without any coaxing from her dad. You'll get started in Phase 6 with negative chin-ups, a slow-motion exercise in which you start with your chin over the bar and then lower yourself. You might be able to do a chin-up by the time you're finished with this book's programs, but more likely it'll take a while longer. (You can repeat Stage 6 if you want to continue working toward a chin-up using your full body weight and no assistance.) The reward? You'll be stronger, pound for pound, than most of the guys in your gym. More important, you'll be able to use your body the way it was designed in a pulling exercise.

Of course, many other muscles are involved in pulls. Your trapezius has a role in pulls from any angle, and the rear parts of your deltoid muscles get involved in most. Your biceps and various forearm muscles also work in concert with your back muscles. On exercises like underhand-grip lat pulldowns and negative chin-ups you'll feel your biceps working directly.

Finally, there's your rotator cuff, a group of four muscles and tendons involved in most upper-body movements. If you follow sports, you hear about them a lot, particularly when a baseball player or tennis star strains or tears one.

It's easy enough to figure out that muscles described with the word "rotator" are involved in rotating something. In this case it's your upper arm, helping it turn forward (internal rotation) or backward (external rotation). The problem is that some of the biggest upper-body muscles are also involved in one of those actions. Your pectorals and latissimus are your body's strongest internal rotators, and there isn't a comparably strong set of muscles involved in external rotation.

There's nothing wrong with your body's design. The internal rotators are strong for a reason, and if you've ever watched a rodeo cowboy wrestle a calf to the ground, you'll understand why. But in the gym, in the interest of building the body's showiest muscles, internal rotators become even stronger, relative to external rotators, than nature intended. Thus, heavy bench presses have been implicated in rotator-cuff injuries.

Overhead lifts, particularly when done overzealously or with poor form, are also linked to pain and suffering, although for different reasons. These lifts can "impinge" the muscles and connective tissues in the vicinity of the shoulder socket, in effect pinching them until they swell up and cry out for help. Any ailment that contains the suffix "itis," such as bursitis or tendinitis, is your body's way of sending a distress signal.

Negative chin-up

GET READY

- Set up a bench or step beneath the chin-up bar.
- Grab the bar with an underhand grip that's just inside shoulder width (you can make the grip wider or narrower if that's more comfortable). You want your grip to be tight here, like the bar is the neck of that third-grade teacher who made fun of your singing voice and tragically ended your musical aspirations. *Throttle* that sucker.
- Jump up so your chin is over the bar, and hold that position.
- You want your body to be straight from your head to your knees.
- If your body sways a bit at first, wait for it to stop before you start the exercise.
- Bend your knees and cross your ankles in back.

DESCEND

- Lower your body as slowly as possible. Resist gravity until your arms are straight—and straight up from your torso.
- Don't allow your body to sway; you want to descend in a straight line, more or less.
- Straighten your legs, so you're standing again on the box or bench.

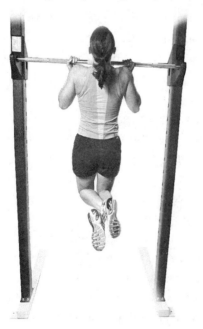 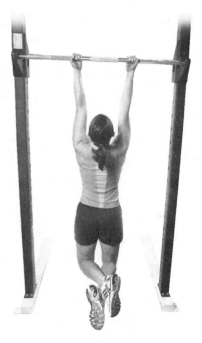

Wide-grip lat pulldown

GET READY

- Attach a long bar to the high pulley of the lat-pulldown machine and select a weight.
- Grab the bar with an overhand grip that's substantially beyond shoulder width.
- Lower yourself to the seat, and position your knees beneath the pad.

LIFT

- Pull the bar down toward your upper chest, squeezing your shoulder blades together in back as you do this. A good mental cue is to imagine that you're pushing your chest out to meet the bar. That prevents the common mistake of rolling the shoulders forward as the lifter pulls the bar down toward her abdomen.

ASCEND

- Slowly allow the bar to rise to the starting position.

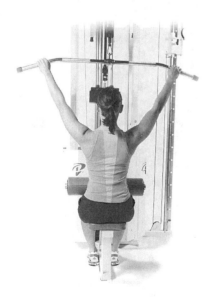
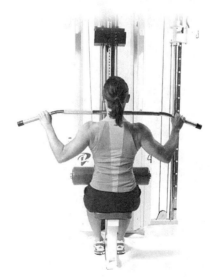

Underhand-grip lat pulldown

GET READY

- Attach any straight bar to the high pulley of the lat-pulldown machine and select a weight.
- Grab the bar with an underhand grip that's about shoulder width, or a bit narrower.
- Position yourself on the seat as described previously.

LIFT

- Pull the bar down toward your upper chest.

ASCEND

- Slowly allow the bar to rise to the starting position.

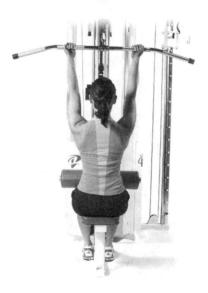 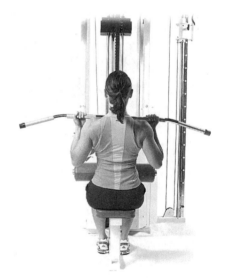

Pullover

This is an alternative exercise for women who work out at home and don't have access to a cable apparatus. It's not a perfect substitute for the lat pulldown, since the muscle-use pattern is different. It still works your lats, but uses them in concert with your pectorals and triceps, instead of with your trapezius and biceps. And since you're lying on your back on a bench, you're partially inhibiting the movements of your shoulder blades.

Ironically, the best version of this exercise is done at a lat-pulldown station (which doesn't help at all with the original problem, i.e., the fact you don't have a lat-pulldown station in your home gym). In that one, you attach a straight bar to the high pulley, stand facing it as you grab it with a wide, overhead grip, and pull it down toward the front of your thighs. You'll feel your lats working in tandem with your pectorals and abdominals. And, unlike the free-weight version, you're resisting gravity throughout the entire range of motion.

But if you're at home, you'll have to make do with the free-weight version.

GET READY
- You can do this with a barbell, an EZ curl bar (that's the one with diagonal indentations near the middle, allowing you to grip the bar in positions that are in between underhand and overhand), or dumbbells. If you choose the latter, you can hold them with your palms facing out or toward each other. There's also a version of the exercise using one dumbbell held in both hands, but it offers no advantages over these.
- Lie on your back on a bench, feet flat on the floor, and hold the weight or weights up over your chest with straight arms.

DESCEND
- Lower the weight(s) straight back behind your head, until your arms are in line with your torso and parallel to the floor.

LIFT
- Pull the weight(s) straight back to the starting position.

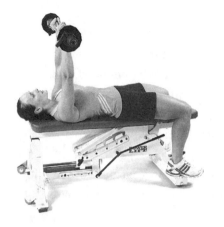

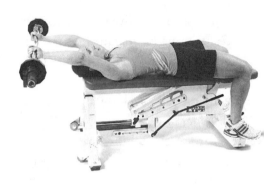

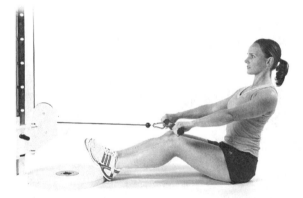

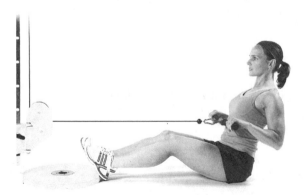

Seated row

GET READY

- Attach a straight bar to the low pulley of the cable-row station and select a weight.
- Grab the bar with an overhand, shoulder-width grip.
- Position yourself on the bench so your feet are against the foot supports, your knees are bent, your torso is upright, your lower back is in its natural arch, and your arms are straight. You should feel tension in the cable at this point.

LIFT

- Pull the bar toward the middle of your abdomen, keeping your shoulders down and feeling your shoulder blades squeeze together in back.

RETURN

- Slowly allow the bar to return to the starting position.

If you work out at home

No cable station? Just substitute a bent-over row for the cable row. You can do any of the versions shown on the following pages, or substitute an underhand-grip bent-over row for variety. You can use a barbell or dumbbells.

Barbell bent-over row

GET READY

- Grab a barbell with an overhand, shoulder-width grip.
- Stand with your feet shoulder-width apart.
- Bend your knees slightly, push your hips back, and bend forward at the hips, keeping the natural arch in your lower back.
- Hold the bar straight down from your shoulders.

LIFT

- Pull the bar to your upper abdomen, keeping your torso and lower body in the same positions.

DESCEND

- Slowly lower the bar to the starting position.

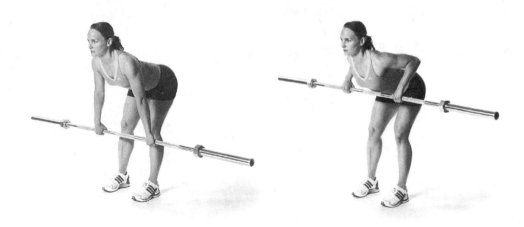

Dumbbell bent-over row

GET READY

- Grab a pair of dumbbells and stand with your feet shoulder-width apart.
- Bend your knees slightly, push your hips back, and bend forward at the hips, keeping the natural arch in your lower back.
- Hold the weights straight down from your shoulders with an overhand (knuckles-out) grip.

LIFT

- Pull the weights straight up to the sides of your abdomen, keeping your torso and lower body in the same positions.

DESCEND

- Slowly lower the weights to the starting position.

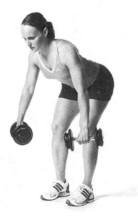 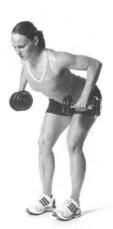

Dumbbell one-point row

GET READY

- Grab a pair of dumbbells.
- Balancing your weight on your left foot, bend forward at the hips and raise your right leg so it forms a T with your torso and your left leg. Your shoulders should be square to the floor.
- Hold the weights at arm's length below your shoulders.

LIFT

- Pull the weights straight up to the sides of your abdomen, keeping your shoulders square to the floor.

DESCEND

- Slowly lower the weights to the starting position.
- Do half the repetitions, then switch legs and finish the set.
- If the set calls for an odd number of reps, round up or down by one rep so you do the same number balancing on each leg. If you end up doing an odd number of reps anyway, start the next set balancing on the leg that got shortchanged.

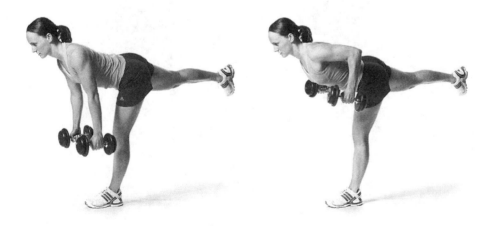

Dumbbell two-point row

GET READY

- Grab a dumbbell and hold it in your nondominant hand with an overhand grip.
- Stand as you would for the standard bent-over row described previously—feet shoulder-width apart, knees bent slightly, hips back, torso bent forward at the hips.
- Hold the weight straight down from your shoulder, with your nonworking hand behind your back.

LIFT

- Pull the weight straight up to the side of your abdomen.

DESCEND

- Lower the weight to the starting position.
- Finish all the reps, then repeat the set with the other arm.

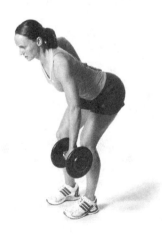 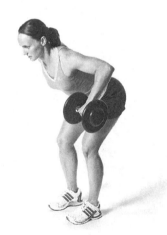

Dumbbell prone Cuban snatch

GET READY

- Set an exercise bench to a low incline (about 30 degrees or less) and grab a pair of dumbbells.
- Lie facedown on the bench, with the dumbbells hanging straight down from your shoulders and your knuckles facing out. (If you were holding a barbell, this would be an overhand grip.)
- You can also kneel on the bench (as our model is doing in the photos), if that works better for you.

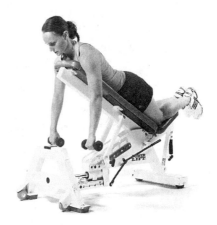

LIFT

- Pull your upper arms up and out to your sides so your upper arms are nearly perpendicular to your torso.
- Allow your elbows to bend, so when your upper arms are on the same plane as your torso, your elbows are bent 90 degrees and your lower arms continue to point down toward the floor.
- Without changing the angle of your upper arms relative to your torso or to the floor, rotate your arms so the weights rise up to about the level of your ears. Make sure your elbows stay bent 90 degrees.

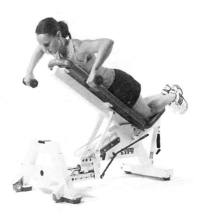

DESCEND

- Lower the weights in the reverse of the two-step sequence—rotate your upper arms so the weights are again pointing toward the floor, then lower them to the starting position.

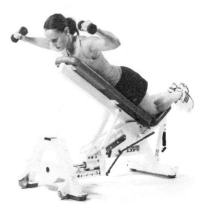

YTWL

Remember the last wedding reception you attended, where the band played "YMCA," and everyone knew how to make the letters with their arms, including your eighty-year-old grandmother and your six-year-old niece? This is exactly the same, only without the music or alcohol, and it's done with weights on a bench instead of standing on the dance floor in a bridesmaid's dress. Okay, it's not even remotely similar, except that you will move your arms in ways that vaguely resemble four letters of the alphabet.

GET READY

- Set an exercise bench to a low incline (about 30 degrees or less) and grab a pair of very light dumbbells.
- Lie facedown on the bench, with the dumbbells hanging straight down from your shoulders.

Y

- Hold the dumbbells in a "neutral" grip (thumbs forward, pinkies back).
- Keeping your arms straight, lift the weights up until your arms and torso form the letter Y. Your thumbs should be up and your pinkies down.
- Slowly lower the weights. Finish the reps and go straight to the T without stopping.

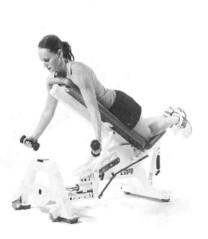
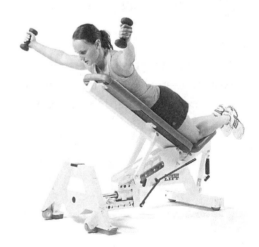

T

- Hold the dumbbells in an underhand grip (pinkies facing each other, thumbs out).
- Keeping your arms straight, lift the weights out to your sides until your arms and torso form the letter T. Your thumbs should be up and your pinkies down.
- Slowly lower the weights. Finish the reps and go straight to the W without stopping.

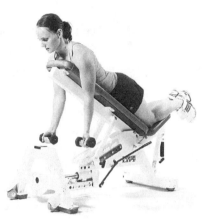

W

- Hold the dumbbells in a neutral grip, with your elbows bent 90 degrees and in close to your torso.
- Rotate your arms up and out. Lead with your thumbs, as if you were hitching a ride in a movie from the 1940s.
- Slowly lower the weights. Finish the reps and go straight to the L without stopping.

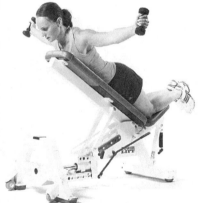

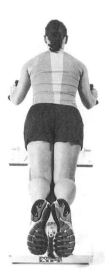
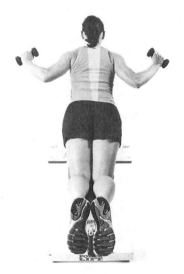

L

- Hold the dumbbells in an overhand grip, with your arms hanging straight down from your shoulders.
- The movement is exactly like the prone Cuban snatch described previously. Pull your arms up until your upper arms are perpendicular to your torso, with your elbows bent 90 degrees.
- Now rotate your upper arms, keeping your elbows bent, until the weights are next to your ears.
- Unlike the Cuban snatch, you'll keep your upper arms in the same position for all your repetitions, rotating up and then slowly rotating back down.
- Finish the reps, then set the weights down and take the designated rest.

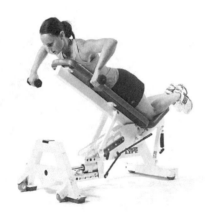 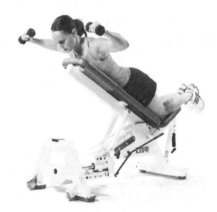

CORE EXERCISES

WHAT THEY ARE These are the exercises I didn't make fun of in Chapter 9.

WHAT MUSCLES THEY WORK The "abdominals" include four sets of muscles. There's the rectus abdominis, of course, which is what ninety-nine percent of us think of when someone mentions "abs." Your external obliques are on the sides of your waist. Beneath them are the internal obliques, and beneath them is the transverse abdominis.

Classic bodybuilding methodology says you're supposed to develop exercises that work the rectus and obliques separately, with really old-school bodybuilders going so far as to use an exercise called the vacuum for the transverse abdominis. (It consists of sucking your belly back toward your spine.)

But the current thinking focuses on movements. Thus, Alwyn includes exercises for three distinct actions: spinal flexion (bringing your ribs down closer to your pelvis), hip flexion (bringing your pelvis up toward your ribs), and side or lateral flexion (pretty much exactly what it sounds like). There's also a fourth movement, back extension, which is the opposite of spinal flexion. It works your spinal erectors, the fibers of which run north and south, like those in your rectus abdominis.

These exercises are, in a way, companions to the YTWL sequence described previously. Those exercises shore up the muscles and connective tissues designed to move and protect your shoulder blades, and these do the same for the muscles between your ribs and pelvis.

Here's another way to look at it: Your body has four "communications centers." The first two are your hips, which act like routers in a computer network. Change the position of your legs, and you change the types of movements that are possible. That's why Alwyn includes so many variations on lunges and step-ups, without any exercises that strictly isolate specific portions of hip movements. With the hips, what's most important is getting the big movements right.

In the other two centers, your middle abdomen and the area between your shoulder blades, many of your circuits of muscle fibers and connective tissue intersect. If anything goes wrong with your shoulders or lower back, those problems will have repercussions from head to toe.

Thus, it's worthwhile to isolate specific muscle actions that affect these muscular crossroads, even if there's nothing about the movements themselves that translates to something you do in real life.

This section is a bit different from the others, in that most of the exercises are shown in sequences. The idea is the same as with the push-ups, shown earlier. You want to do the most challenging variation possible, given the parameters of the individual workouts. You don't have to start with the first variation of the plank or Swiss-ball crunch, if you're already able to do a more advanced version. (You need to do the side-flexion series in order, for reasons that will become apparent when you try the first part. I speak from experience when I say it's harder than it looks.) And you may need to go back and forth, doing one version for higher-rep workouts and another when the workout calls for lower reps.

What's most important is that the exercises never feel "easy"; you should always feel as if you're challenging your body to get stronger.

PLANK EXERCISES

45-degree plank

GET READY

- Place your forearms on a padded exercise bench, and balance your weight on your forearms and toes, with your body at a 45-degree angle to the floor.
- Align your body so it forms a straight line from your ankles through your neck.

HOLD

- Hold that position for the time indicated in the workout chart.

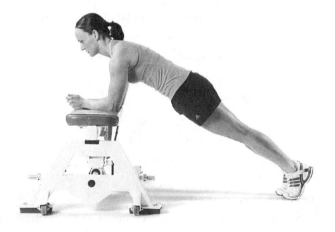

Plank

GET READY

- Set a mat on the floor, or find a well-padded area to rest your forearms.
- Place your forearms on the floor, and balance your weight on your forearms and toes.
- Align your body so it forms a straight line from your ankles through your neck.

HOLD:

- Hold that position for the time indicated in the workout chart.

Swiss-ball plank

GET READY

- Snag a Swiss ball and set it up alongside an exercise bench.
- Set the balls of your feet on the bench and your forearms on the ball.
- Carefully maneuver the ball away from the bench until you're able to stretch out into the plank position, with your weight balanced on your forearms and toes and your body forming a straight line from your ankles through your neck.

HOLD:

- Hold that position for the time indicated.

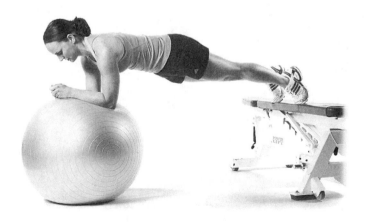

Three-point Swiss-ball plank

GET READY

- Get into plank position with your forearms on the Swiss ball and your feet on the bench, as described previously.
- Lift one foot off the bench and into the air, keeping your body in the same alignment.

HOLD:

- Hold that position for half the time indicated, then switch legs for the remainder.

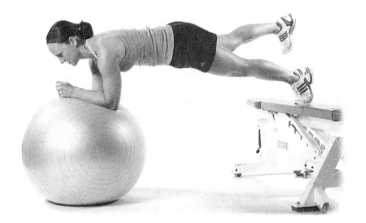

HIP FLEXION EXERCISES

Prone jackknife

GET READY

- Grab a Swiss ball and set your shins on top of it, with your palms flat on the floor.
- Carefully walk your palms out until your body is in push-up position, forming a straight line from your ankles through your neck.

LIFT

- Pull your knees toward your chest, allowing your torso to shift diagonally so your hips rise toward the ceiling and your head tilts down toward the floor.
- Keep your arms straight, and your neck in line with your torso.
- Your toes will end up on top of the ball, with most of your weight now shifted to your hands.

RETURN

- Roll the ball back to the starting position, so your shins are again on top of the ball and your body is aligned from ankles to neck.

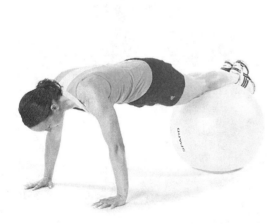 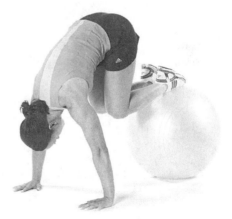

Reverse crunch

GET READY

- Lie on your back on the floor, with your arms at your sides, palms on the floor, and hips and knees bent about 90 degrees.

LIFT

- Contract your abdominal muscles and pull your thighs up toward your ribs.

RETURN

- Lower your legs to the starting position.

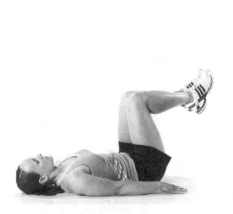 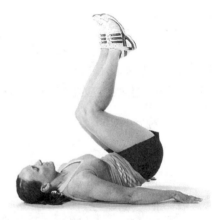

Incline reverse crunch

GET READY

- Set up an incline bench to whatever angle allows you to challenge yourself for the suggested number of reps.
- Lie on your back on the bench, and grab on to the bench however you can (it varies from person to person and from bench to bench).
- Start with your feet off the floor and your hips and knees bent at 90-degree angles.

LIFT

- Contract your abdominal muscles and pull your thighs up toward your ribs.

RETURN

- Lower your legs to the starting position.

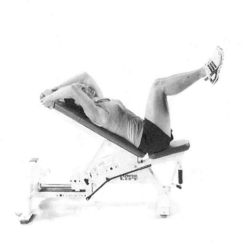
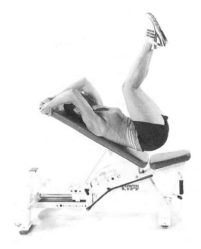

SWISS-BALL CRUNCH VARIATIONS

Swiss-ball crunch

GET READY

- Lie on your back on a Swiss ball so your body forms a straight line from your ears through your shoulders, torso, thighs, and knees.
- Set your feet firmly on the ground, with your knees bent about 90 degrees and your legs open just enough to provide a stable platform and prevent you from rolling sideways off the ball.
- Fold your arms across your chest, or, for a greater challenge, place your hands behind your ears (as shown).
- Tighten your hamstrings and gluteals.

LIFT

- Keeping your hips up and your hamstrings and gluteals tight, contract your abdominal muscles as you lift your shoulders and pull your ribs toward your pelvis.

DESCEND

- Lower your torso back to the starting position.

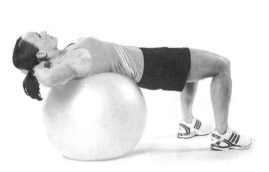 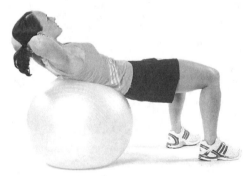

Weighted Swiss-ball crunch

GET READY

- Grab a weight plate or dumbbell, and lie on your back on a Swiss ball, as described previously.
- Hold the weight across your chest.

LIFT

- Contract your abdominal muscles as you lift your shoulders and pull your ribs toward your pelvis.

DESCEND

- Lower your torso back to the starting position.

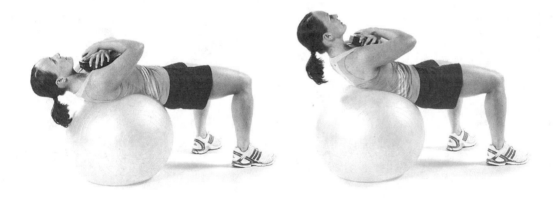

Long-arm Swiss-ball crunch

GET READY

- Lie on your back on a Swiss ball, as described previously.
- Extend your arms back behind your head so your fingers touch.

LIFT

- Contract your abdominal muscles as you lift your shoulders and pull your ribs toward your pelvis.

DESCEND

- Lower your torso back to the starting position.

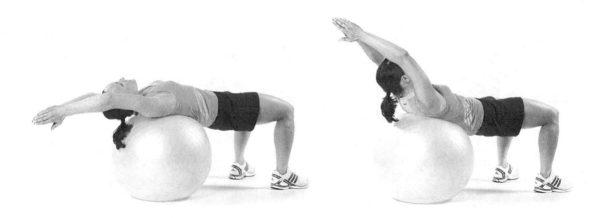

Infinite quest

You can make this progressively more challenging by holding objects of differing sizes and weights behind your head. Every time you move your hands and shift the center of gravity, you give your midbody muscles something different to do. You can start by holding a light medicine ball, for example, and progress to holding something big and awkward, like another Swiss ball. (Yes, it'll look goofy as heck, but I guarantee you'll feel the difference.)

You can also play with different weights—a single weight plate or dumbbell held in both hands, two dumbbells with your hands apart, a light barbell . . .

The variety is infinite, but you have to pay attention to your body. If you feel a strain in your neck, shoulders, or upper back, stop the set, and try an easier variation.

LATERAL FLEXION EXERCISES

Hanna side flexion 1

GET READY

- Lie on your right side, with your legs on top of each other and bent 90 degrees at the hips and knees. Your upper legs are perpendicular to your torso.
- Your elbows are near your ears, with your hands touching behind your head and your right upper arm flat on the floor and supporting your head.
- You want your body to form a straight line from your nose through your belly button to the middle of your pelvis. It's like the starting position for the reverse crunch, described earlier, but on your side instead of your back.

LIFT

- Rotate your left thigh so your left lower leg rises above your right leg, forming a 45-degree angle, more or less.
- Hold that position for a count of five.

DESCEND

- Lower your leg slowly, do all your repetitions at the same deliberate speed, and then switch sides and repeat the set.

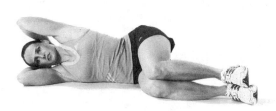 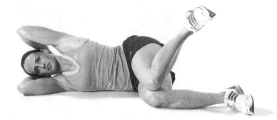

Hanna side flexion 2

GET READY

- Lie on your right side, as described for side flexion 1.

LIFT

- Keeping your legs in place, raise your head and upper torso toward your left hip.
- Hold for 5 seconds.

DESCEND

- Lower your head and torso slowly, do all your repetitions at the same deliberate speed, and then switch sides and repeat the set.

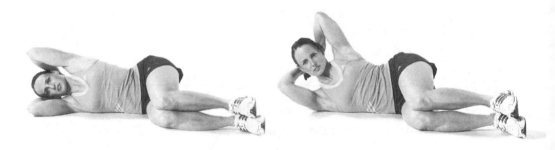

Hanna side flexion 3

GET READY

- Lie on your right side, as described for side flexion 1.

LIFT

- Lift your head and torso toward your left hip, as in side flexion 2, while at the same time rotating your left leg upward as you did in side flexion 1.
- Hold for 5 seconds.

DESCEND

- Lower your head, torso, and leg slowly and simultaneously, do all your repetitions at the same deliberate speed, and then switch sides and repeat the set.

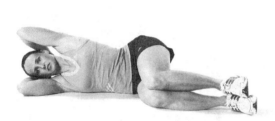
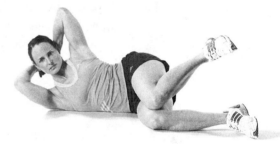

Swiss-ball side crunch

GET READY

- Grab a Swiss ball and set it up near a wall.
- Lie on your right side on the ball, with your left leg over your right and both feet braced against the bottom of the wall.
- Hold your hands behind your ears.

LIFT

- Contract your oblique muscles on your left side as you lift your head and shoulders and crunch your ribs down toward your left hip.

DESCEND

- Slowly return to the starting position.
- Finish all your reps, then repeat the set lying on your left side on the ball, with your right leg over your left.

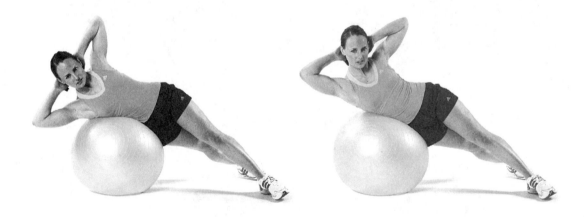

TWISTING EXERCISES

Cable horizontal wood chop

GET READY

- Attach a rope handle to an adjustable cable pulley that's set at midbody height.
- Grab the rope with both hands, and stand with your right side to the weight stack, about three feet away from the stack.
- Set your feet shoulder-width apart, bend your knees slightly, and turn your shoulders to the right so you're holding the rope just outside the right side of your torso.

LIFT

- Pull the rope across your torso in a horizontal line, turning your shoulders so the rope ends up past the left side of your torso.
- Follow the rope with your eyes all the way, and keep your head and shoulders aligned, so they turn as a unit.

DESCEND

- Reverse the sequence as you return to the starting position.
- Finish all the reps, then switch sides and repeat the set.

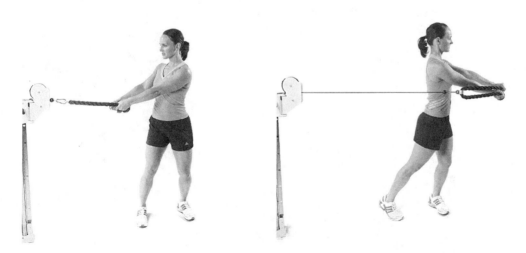

Home-gym alternative (not shown): You can lie on your back on the floor, with knees bent and feet flat on the floor, and pull a dumbbell, medicine ball, or any other weighted object along the same trajectory. For a greater challenge, you can do this lying on a Swiss ball.

Reverse wood chop

GET READY

- Attach a rope handle to a low cable pulley.
- Grab the rope with both hands, and stand with your right side to the weight stack, about three feet away from the stack.
- Set your feet shoulder-width apart, push your hips back slightly, and turn your shoulders to the right so you're holding the rope just outside your right knee.

LIFT

- Pull the rope up across your torso in a diagonal line, straightening your knees and hips and turning your shoulders so the rope ends up just past and above your left shoulder.
- Follow the rope with your eyes all the way, and keep your head and shoulders aligned, so they turn as a unit.

DESCEND

- Reverse the sequence as you return to the starting position.
- Finish all the reps, then switch sides and repeat the set.

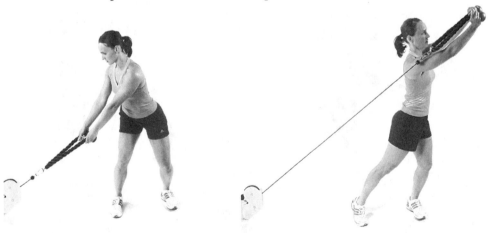

Home-gym alternative (not shown): You can lift a dumbbell, medicine ball, or any weighted object along the same trajectory.

BACK-EXTENSION EXERCISES

Back extension (not shown)

GET READY

- Position yourself on the back-extension apparatus so your heels are under the rear pads and the front of your pelvis rests on the bigger front pad.
- Set your body in a straight line from your neck to your ankles.
- You can fold your arms across your chest, or set your fingers behind your ears for a greater challenge.

DESCEND

- Bend forward at the hips—not at the waist—and go down as far as you can without losing the natural arch in your lower back.

LIFT

- Squeeze your gluteals as you pull your torso back up to the starting position. You should feel this in your hamstrings and gluteals, which are the working parts. Your lower back has to work to hold its natural shape and support your spine, but the muscles in that area should only be working isometrically, not going through a range of motion.

Advanced version: Try it holding a weight plate across your chest.

Home-gym alternative: Do the prone cobra, described next, if you don't have access to a back-extension apparatus.

Prone cobra

GET READY

- Lie facedown on a mat or well-padded floor.
- Your hands are at your sides, palms up, and your forehead should touch the floor. The tops of your feet should be as flat against the floor as you can get them.

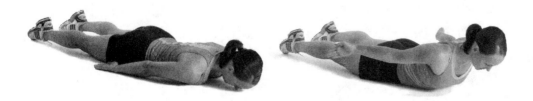

LIFT

- Slowly lift your head and shoulders off the floor, rotating your arms to the out-side until your thumbs are pointing up.
- Squeeze your shoulder blades together in back, and hold for the time designated in the workout chart.

DESCEND

- Slowly lower yourself to the floor.

BODY-WEIGHT MATRIX

These exercises are used in phases 3 and 5 at the end of Workout A.

Squat

This is simply a body-weight version of the classic exercise. Hold your hands up near your ears, and do your twenty-four squats quickly without sacrificing form.

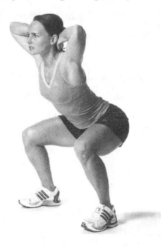

Lunge

Again, this is simply the body-weight version of the exercise. Hold your hands up near your ears, and do 12 reps with each leg, alternating as you go (right-left-right-left, etc.).

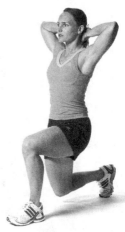

Lunge jump

Instead of alternating legs by stepping forward and back, you'll jump up from each lunge and switch legs in midair, then descend into the next lunge upon landing. Go for a smooth, continuous series of jumps and lunges, twelve with each leg. You aren't trying to move forward as you do them; do them all in the same spot.

Squat jump

As with the lunge jumps, you'll jump up from each squat, then descend immediately into the next squat and jump. Try to get up in the air on all twenty-four jumps.

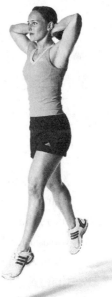

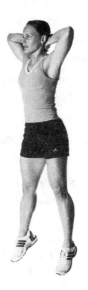

Extra Stuff to Do*

Alwyn's programs in Chapter 10 call for two or three workouts a week. With fewer than two workouts, you won't get the results the programs are designed to elicit. With more than three, you won't recover enough between workouts to get the benefits you want. Your body will quickly become overtrained, and at that point the *best* you can hope for is that you make no improvements in strength or muscle size. The worst is that you lose strength and muscle size. You also might find yourself battling constant colds and infections, having trouble sleeping, and experiencing the other problems I mentioned in Chapter 7 as signs that you aren't eating enough.

If you remember nothing else from this penultimate chapter, I want you to memorize this phrase, which comes directly from Alwyn: "You don't get better by training. You get better by *recovering* from training." Your goal is to give your body the right stimulus—serious exercise—and then give it time to adapt to that stimulus.

---

*I got this phrase from Mark Verstegen, author of *Core Performance,* on which I worked as an editor. "Extra Stuff to Do" is a play on ESD, an abbreviation for "energy-systems development." That's the technical phrase for what most of us would call "cardio." Mark, like Alwyn and most of the really smart physical-performance specialists today, maintains a healthy skepticism about doing endurance exercise for its own sake.

Most of us think of recovery, if we think about it at all, as allowing muscles time to refuel and repair themselves between workouts. And that's perfectly accurate, as far as it goes. What gets tricky is figuring out all the factors that might alter the formula.

I've been working out with weights since I was thirteen, and at fifty, I'm still learning what my body can and can't do. When stress in my life is relatively low, I can do three hard workouts a week, and sometimes I'll throw in a fourth workout, if it's possible on the program I'm doing at the time. When stress is high (like, say, a few days before my deadline on this book), I'm happy to get in two workouts, and I don't even think about pushing myself to my limits.

Never forget, you're the CEO of your body, as well as its sole employee. You have to determine your goals and simultaneously manage the workload necessary to reach those goals.

With that said, let's look at a few types of exercise and physical activity you might consider adding to the *New Rules* workouts.

ENDURANCE EXERCISE

At the end of Chapter 3, I wrote about a system Alwyn has used to combine intervals with more traditional steady-pace endurance work. You'd do fifteen to twenty minutes of intervals (one minute of hard running or riding, followed by a two-minute recovery period of easier running or riding), then come to a complete stop for five minutes. Then you'd run or ride at a steady, comfortable speed for however long you want.

This technique isn't prescribed as any mandatory part of the workouts. But you're welcome to try it on the days between weight workouts, if you want, with one precaution:

You'll note that several workouts detailed in Chapter 10 include intervals at the end—Stage 2, Workout B, for example. *Do not* do the interval/steady-state combo the day after one of those workouts.

This leaves you with two choices:

- You can do the workout as designed, with the intervals, and then wait a day before doing the interval/steady-state combo. You can then take another day off, or lift the following day. (Alwyn never includes intervals in consecutive workouts.)
- You can skip the intervals following the weight workout, and do the interval/

steady-state combo the following day. Then you can either take the following day off (which I recommend), or do the next weight workout as designed.

What about traditional endurance exercise in between weight workouts?

Again, it's up to you. I'm not your father, your boss, or your coach. I'm just a bald-headed guy who writes books. You're free to do as much or as little as you want.

My only caution is that high volumes of endurance exercise—training for a marathon, for example—would be counterproductive. There's just no point in trying to make your body smaller and more efficient at the same time you're trying to make it stronger and rev up your metabolism.

YOGA AND PILATES

My gut tells me that Pilates and most types of yoga would be good complements to a serious strength-training program. You'd certainly fulfill the first requirement for recovery: Don't make it worse. Both yoga and Pilates have been linked to improvements in chronic lower-back pain, which suggests to me that they wouldn't produce the kind of muscle damage that would hinder your progress.

Still, I don't know of any research that's addressed the compatibility of strength training and yoga or Pilates.

Friends of mine in the yogic-American community assure me that the quality of the instructor matters. My wife, who's tortured by a variety of upper- and lower-back problems (in addition to the pain in the neck she married), sometimes returns from yoga class feeling worse instead of better. Some instructors are good at helping participants with correct form on difficult poses, and some push them too far, or fail to correct problems.

The clear and obvious benefit of these exercise systems, it seems to me, is that you get blood into the muscles you worked in the weight room. With blood comes heat and nutrients, and both should help those muscles recover.

But there's also a potential drawback to yoga (which doesn't really apply to Pilates). Women tend to be more flexible than men, which is usually seen as an advantage. But the greater the range of motion in your joints, the softer and more pliable your connective tissues tend to be. The degree of stiffness in those tissues tends to determine their injury risk. More stiffness means more protection from injury. More laxity means more chance that something can go wrong.

So, while yoga is usually associated with positive health outcomes, it also produces greater flexibility, and for some people, too much is as bad as too little.

SPINNING, BOOT CAMP, KICKBOXING, AND SPORT-SPECIFIC CLASSES

On the bright side, these workouts can encourage recovery from serious weight lifting, in that they help you heat up your muscles while flooding them with nutrient-rich blood. The downside is that they're all variations on interval training, and because of the way gyms like to schedule things, they're usually forty-five minutes to an hour long.

That's a hellaciously long time to do intervals, especially when you're already challenging yourself in two or three weight workouts a week.

So my advice is to put a day in between one of these classes and any weight workout that includes intervals. Here's an example of how that could work:

	Monday	Tuesday	Wednesday	Thursday	Friday	Saturday
Week 1	Weight workout, no intervals	Spinning	Off	Weight workout with intervals	Yoga, Pilates, easy endurance exercise, or off	Weight workout, no intervals
Week 2	Weight workout, with intervals	Off	Kickboxing	Weight workout, no intervals	Yoga, Pilates, easy endurance exercise, or off	Weight workout, with intervals

In this example, Sunday is always a complete day of rest, and you have one or two recovery days during the week. You also manage your use of intervals by putting at least one day in between similarly challenging workouts.

SUPPLEMENTAL STRENGTH TRAINING

There's a particular type of lifter who'll look at a workout and immediately try to improve upon it by adding exercises for a particular part of the body. "There's no direct work for my biceps. So I'll just add some curls. And maybe some kickbacks for my triceps. And maybe some lateral raises for my shoulders . . ." It goes on and on, until the workout looks more like the inbred child of *Shape* and *Flex* magazines than anything a veteran coach like Alwyn would design.

My advice: Stop the temptation to "improve" the workouts before it starts. If you need to work around orthopedic problems, that's different. If you have a medical condition that calls for modifications, again, you're encouraged to make whatever changes you need, preferably with professional guidance.

But if you're tempted to tinker with these workouts for the sake of doing more for something that, on paper, appears to be neglected, all I can say is, "Don't." These workouts are balanced, and they've been tested and refined by thousands of women trained by Alwyn and his staff over the years.

HIKING, BACKPACKING, HEAVY-DUTY LANDSCAPING, OR HOME REMODELING

It may not look or even feel like serious exercise—you aren't, after all, doing sets or reps or listening to an instructor tell you when to change speeds. But an hours-long hike or a Saturday spent planting your garden can wear you out in ways you don't anticipate. A day working a shovel and rake may put unusual strain on your lower back, or leave you with blistered hands and exhausted forearms. A few hours hanging drywall can do a number on your upper back and shoulders. A hike in the great outdoors might be so exhilarating that you don't even notice how deeply you've exhausted every muscle in your lower body. (Although you'll probably notice the next day.)

You certainly aren't training for anything when you hike or move furniture or plant azaleas. But your body doesn't know that. It just knows it's exhausted, and it's most likely worn out in such a unique way that it could take days of recovery before you're ready for a serious workout.

There's no rule for when you can get back to your regular workout schedule after a tiring day in the yard or on the trail. The key is to realize that you've just done something that requires recovery. How much you need can only be determined by you.

BUSINESS TRIPS AND VACATIONS

I'm continually surprised by how many readers ask me vacation-related questions every spring and summer. My first instinct is to say, "Enjoy yourself and don't stress over taking a week or two off from formal workouts."

But, to be honest, I don't follow that advice.

I like to work out, and I often squeeze in workouts when and where I can. Still, I don't try to do the workouts in the particular program I'm following at the time.

If I'm working out in a big, commercial gym (most will allow visitors to pay a day rate to work out), I'll mess around with equipment I don't typically get to use. If I'm in a bare-bones facility, like a hotel gym, I'll challenge myself to make up exercises that give me a complete workout despite the lack of equipment. My goal is to have fun, test my creativity, and not do anything stupid that spoils my business trip or vacation.

Another consideration is stress management. If squeezing in a workout relieves your stress, then it's a good idea. (Yeah, like you needed me to tell you that.) But if it adds to your stress, and you're doing it only because you feel you have to, then it might be a better idea to take care of business first (on vacation, your job is to have fun and enjoy whatever company you have) and save the workouts for when you return to your real life.

DIMINISHING RETURNS

With any type of exercise, there's a point at which you're doing more harm than good. You can probably tell if you're reaching that point by asking yourself this simple question: "Do I really feel like doing yoga tonight?" (Or Spinning, or kickboxing, or whatever you feel obligated to do aside from your weight workouts.) If the answer is yes, and it's an honest yes, then it's unlikely you're pushing yourself too far. But if you ask that question and realize you'd rather do almost anything else, then you probably should save your energy for a future workout.

Fitness geeks like me talk about the importance of listening to your body, but sometimes it's just as important to listen to your brain. Sagging motivation tends to be a pretty good sign that you're trying to do too much.

Personally, the older I get, the more I pay attention to my motivation. If I really want to hit the weights, but for some reason have to skip that day's workout, I get cranky. (Others might say I turn into a turbo-powered jerk. I admit I'm not the best judge of my attitude when I'm workout-deprived.) But if the opposite happens, and I work out despite feeling sluggish and unmotivated, I tend to come down with something—a cold, sinus infection, or whatever the kids bring home from school that week.

Final thought on this subject:

Remember that your gym, no matter how clean and well maintained, is still a launching pad for whatever viruses are going around. And, if anything, the viruses are more motivated than you are.

All it takes is for one person to enter the place bearing a communicable disease—the employee who swipes your card at the front desk, the yoga instructor who uses her hands to correct your form, or the chatty woman sharing the lat-pulldown station—and chances are good you'll be exposed to whatever she has. If your defenses are in any way compromised because of exhaustion, undernutrition, stress, or the fact your body's already trying to fight off a rival virus, you could be in worse shape than if you'd put the workout aside for another day.

Yes, You

NEW RULE #21 • The biggest blocks to your success could be the ones you've erected

Almost every day, I get a certain kind of e-mail:

> I just bought [*New Rules of Lifting* / *Book of Muscle* / *Home Workout Bible* / *Testosterone Advantage Plan*] and I [liked it / loved it / filed a class-action lawsuit to prevent you from ever writing another workout book]. I've been telling all my friends to [buy it / avoid it / know that Jesus loves them]. I have just [one question / two questions / three questions / one rambling monologue]:
>
> I [do yoga three times a week / want to start training for a marathon / am irresistible to fire ants]. So I was wondering if I should [do the programs as written in your book / don't do the programs as written in your book / move to Thailand]. Or should I [do something different / return the book for a refund / ask Oprah's trainer]?

By the way, I should mention that I [work out in a home gym that consists of one 10-pound dumbbell, a Swiss ball that leaks, and one rusty coffee can filled with marbles / tend to fall asleep with heavy weights in my hands / have three weeks to live].

I don't mean to make fun of anyone's medical condition or personal issues. But I am continually amazed at the idea many of us have that our minor roadblocks present uniquely Herculean obstacles. I include myself in that category, by the way. Back in 1990, I was working as a feature writer at a newspaper that went out of business. I was distraught, and asked one of the paper's top editors what I should do.

"Get another job," he advised.

"But where else would I fit in?" I asked.

He stared at me for a moment. "Any place that needs a feature writer."

I saw myself as a unique talent, someone who could only be valued and productive under special, planet-aligning circumstances. He saw me as someone he'd hired because he thought I could do the job better than the other applicants. Since I hadn't done anything to convince him otherwise, he didn't see why the next editor who needed a feature writer wouldn't view me the same way.

This brings me all the way back to something I wrote in the introduction:

"What I can't bring myself to do is find a hundred ways to say 'you can do it!' You can do it if you want to do it. I know it. You know it. Do I really need to say it over and over?"

I've corresponded with countless readers over the years, and I find myself sorting them into two camps. There's the group that, in my view, wants to succeed in their workout program, however they might define success. And there's the group that wants me to help them validate their excuses for not succeeding.

Unfair? Sure. I probably misjudge people every single day. But when you do what I do as long as I've done it, you start to see some patterns. And one pattern immediately sets off alarm bells in my mind: If the first words in my correspondent's question present some sort of excuse for not following through with the programs, I'll assume he or she will never follow through on the advice I give, no matter how good or bad it may be.

I'll give you two examples:

If a guy approaches me about losing his gut, but makes it clear he has no plans to stop drinking beer, I assume there's no way I can help him. I simply don't know how a beer drinker can lose a beer belly unless he stops drinking beer.

If a woman approaches me about doing a workout program that requires exercise equipment, but tells me she won't join a gym and won't get the equipment she needs to work out at home, I assume she doesn't really want to do the program. Again, I can't tell someone how to do a workout program without equipment when the exercises very plainly call for equipment.

There's a clear path from where they are to where they say they want to be. But there's just as clear a roadblock they've installed that prevents them from following that path.

I don't mean to say that there's no such thing as a genuine obstacle that calls for professional advice. I also get plenty of e-mails from readers who need help working around injuries or scheduling nightmares. I've brainstormed with religiously observant readers about how to make it through periods of fasting without losing hard-earned strength and muscle size. To the best of my ability, I try to help anyone who seems sincere and prepared to make an effort. Frankly, I'm flattered that anyone even thinks to ask me some of the questions I get asked, which assume levels of expertise that far exceed my actual knowledge and abilities.

Then there's the other kind.

So let me say this about motivation, at the risk of coming off like an anti-self-help guru:

It has to come from inside you. Nobody can give you motivation.

Which brings me to the trickiest problem of all: efficacy. That is, the belief that you can or can't succeed.

I used to work with a woman who was quite overweight. She got weight-loss surgery, it was successful, and one day I saw her in a gym, working with a trainer. She had a look of wonder in her eyes as the trainer showed her how to do a series of basic exercises. Afterward, she told me something that caught me by surprise: "I had never considered myself someone who could exercise."

Not "someone who enjoyed exercise" or "someone who could stick with an exercise program." She simply didn't think that she, as an overweight, nonathletic woman, was physically capable of performing exercise.

That was several years ago, and I've thought a lot about what she said. I don't think there's ever been a day in my life in which I looked at a sport or type of exercise and said, "I can't do that." I've certainly looked at great athletes and realized I couldn't do things as well as they can do them. And there are times when I've chosen not to try something because I didn't think the risk-benefit ratio was solidly in my favor. But to rule out all exercise because of a vague sense that I wasn't capable of doing it? It would never occur to me to think that way.

In other words, my lack of empathy comes from a genuine place: I don't like to think of life as a series of activities I "can" or "can't" do. To me, it's much more useful to see the world as a series of choices. There are some things I choose to do (work, exercise, follow my favorite baseball team) and things I choose not to do (learn a foreign language, hunt and fish, play online poker).

Sure, there are things at which I would surely fail if I attempted them. I couldn't become a professional golfer or Olympic weight lifter no matter how sincerely I chose to pursue those goals. But I can choose to play golf, and I can choose to do Olympic-style weight lifting in the gym. I can choose to get better at either or both of those things. I just can't choose to attain a level of success that my genetics and resources wouldn't allow.

Most of our choices fall between those extremes. There's a world of difference, for example, between choosing to follow a regular workout program with the goal of getting into better shape, and choosing to become a size 0 runway model. If Giorgio Armani has said he'd hire you if you just weighed 5 pounds less, okay, then the latter is a choice you can make. (I hope you wouldn't make that choice, but then again I'm not a fan of runway models.) But for most everyone else, the first choice is realistic, while the second is absurd.

Suppose, however, that you told your friends and coworkers that your goal this year is to fit into your skinny jeans, a goal that probably involves losing 5 to 10 pounds of fat. And suppose there's no physical, medical, or psychiatric reason why you can't reach this goal—you aren't being held hostage and force-fed Ben & Jerry's, your thyroid gland is in good working order, and you aren't one of those people who gets into her car to drive to the gym and ends up in Bolivia.

Since you've made this choice to lose fat knowing full well you're capable of following through, will you? If you're reading this page, you've probably bought the book, which is a good first step. (Thank you, by the way.) Following the training routines and diet plans will clearly help you reach your goal. But making adjustments as you go along—tweaking your diet, occasionally adding to or subtracting from your workout schedule to keep your energy and enthusiasm up—is also part of that choice.

If you've truly made the choice to reach this goal, then you have to act on it whenever it's appropriate. You have to be both systematic and flexible. The flexible part happens when you have to skip a workout or indulge in a "cheat" meal to accommodate the other choices you've made—to be in a relationship, to keep a job, to raise children, to remember the taste of chocolate cake.

But it's the systematic part that defines the choice you've made. You might stumble, you might veer, you might even hit a brick wall at some point. But in the end, if the goal you've articulated is truly a choice and not a daydream or fantasy, then you'll figure out the right system. It's fine to get advice. It's okay to make adjustments and accommodations. It's even all right to change your goal, if you decide your original target is too modest or ambitious.

The choice is yours.

One last thing: Remember that job I lost back in 1990? It took me a couple of years and a series of stumbles, veers, and headlong crashes into brick walls. Then, in 1992, I got a job that I loved even more than the one I'd lost two years before, writing about some of my favorite subjects—exercise, health, and nutrition. I confess I'd never made it a goal to write about those subjects, but that's just because I had no idea anyone could make a living that way. But, because I chose to keep writing, and never backed away from that choice despite a long history of setbacks and screw-ups, I was ready for the opportunity when it came along.

Which brings me back to you. Whether you're a fitness buff, a semi-regular exerciser, or an absolute beginner, the choices you make now will define the opportunities that come up later. Nobody can choose to be perfect, but all of us can choose to be better.

So what's your choice?

Notes

Chapter 1

Fear of straightening elbows: I've seen the precaution in a variety of books and magazines, but only marked this one for future reference. For the record, the sentence I quote is on page 166 of *Body for Life for Women.* I feel guilty picking on Dr. Peeke, since her book has a lot of good advice; it's only because of my shortsighted stupidity that I'm left with just one example at my fingertips.

Mr. Pot, meet Mr. Kettle: As long as I'm making fun of magazines that promise readers results based on physical archetypes—that a woman can look like a dancer if she does a dancer's workout, for example—I should note that I've been guilty of this. In the first chapter of my first book, *The Testosterone Advantage Plan,* my coauthors and I make the point that most guys reading our book would rather look like Olympic sprinters than champion marathoners. Fair enough. But we use that point to argue against the benefits of endurance exercise, implying that aerobic exercise makes you look weak and sickly while anaerobic work—lifting and sprinting—makes you look like someone who "had sex five times before breakfast." Not cool. Not cool at all.

Chapter 2

Gender differences: This information comes from a variety of sources, including *All About Muscle* (Demos, 2000) by Irwin Siegel, M.D., and *Essentials of Strength Training and Conditioning,* the textbook used by the National Strength and Conditioning Association.

Strength and mortality: Rantonen et al., "Handgrip strength and cause-specific and all-cause mortality in older disabled women: exploring the mechanism." *Journal of the American Geriatric Society* 2003 May; 51(5):636–641. Newman et al., "Strength, but not muscle mass, is associated with mortality in the health, aging and body composition study cohort." *Journals of Gerontology Series A: Biological Sciences and Medical Sciences Online* 2006 Jan; 61(1):72–77.

Women should train like men: Lewis et al., "Physiological differences between genders: implications for sports conditioning." *Sports Medicine* 1986; 3:357–369. Holloway and Baechle, "Strength training for female athletes: a review of selected aspects." *Sports Medicine* 1990; 9(4):216–228.

Muscle quality: I borrowed heavily here from *Designing Resistance Training Programs (DRTP),* third edition, by Steven Fleck and William Kraemer. (You'll see a lot of Dr. Kraemer's studies cited in this book, and the fact he runs the exercise physiology program at the University of Connecticut, where Cassandra is getting her Ph.D., has nothing to do with it.)

Muscle gain, fat loss, circumference changes: I used a bunch of different sources, including *DRTP* and an article from *Pure Power* magazine (September 2003) called "Big Iron for the Boys . . . and Girls," by James Krieger.

I saw Dr. Kraemer's MRIs at a scientific conference. They were used to illustrate data from this study: Kraemer et al., "Changes in muscle hypertrophy in women with periodized resistance training." *Medicine & Science in Sports & Exercise* 2004; 36(4):697–708.

Muscle fibers in men and women: Staron et al., "Fiber type composition of the vastus lateralis muscle of young men and women." *The Journal of Histochemistry & Cytochemistry* 2000; 48(5):623–629.

Muscle recovery in men versus women: Esbjornsson-Liljedahl et al., "Smaller muscle ATP reduction in women than in men by repeated bouts of sprint exercise." *Journal of Applied Physiology* 2002; 93:1075–1083.

Muscle soreness in men versus women: Dannecker et al., "Sex differences in delayed onset muscle pain." *Clinical Journal of Pain* 2005; 21:120–126.

Women and muscle inflammation: Peake et al., "Characterization of inflammatory responses to eccentric exercise in humans." *Exercise Immunology Review* 2005; 11:64–85.

Chapter 3

Aerobics: I used a paperback version of *Aerobics;* the excerpted sentences are found in Chapter 3, page 15. I'm not sure when it was published; if that narrows it down, the price on the cover is one dollar.

Calorie calculations: Like everyone who writes about exercise, I calculate calorie burn rates with a chart called "Compendium of Physical Activities," which was originally presented in *Medicine & Science in Sports & Exercise.* It assigns virtually anything you might be doing at any moment a metabolic value, or MET, which tells you how hard the activity is as a multiple of your resting metabolic rate. So "lying quietly and watching television" is a 1 MET activity, as is "sitting on toilet." (Yes, somebody measured this.) I used 1.8 for general work-related activities like word processing. Walking 4 mph is 4 METs. Once you know how many METs an activity is, you multiply it by your weight in kilograms (1 kilogram equals 2.2 pounds). That tells you how many calories you burn in an hour doing that activity. Strenuous weight lifting is 6 METs, as I show in the sidebar at the end of Chapter 3.

Afterburn calculations: I got these from a variety of studies summarized in an article in the November/December 2004 issue of *IDEA Fitness Journal.* The article, titled "Exercise After-Burn: A Research Update," was written by my friend Len Kravitz, Ph.D., and Chantal Vella, Ph.D., his colleague at the University of New Mexico.

Post-workout fat oxidation: Petitt et al., "Effect of resistance exercise on postprandial lipemia." *Journal of Applied Physiology* 2003; 94:694–700.

Elevated resting metabolic rates: Osterberg and Melby, "Effect of acute resistance exercise on postexercise oxygen consumption and resting metabolic rate in young women." *International Journal of Sport Nutrition & Exercise Metabolism* 2000; 10(1):71–81. Lemmer et al., "Effect of strength training on resting metabolic rate and physical activity: age and gender comparisons." *Medicine & Science in Sports & Exercise* 2001; 33(4):532–541.

Increased exercise efficiency with weight loss: Keim et al., "Energy expenditure and physical performance in overweight women: response to training with and without caloric restriction." *Metabolism* 1990; 39(6):651–658.

Shrinking muscle fibers: This, again, is from Drs. Kraemer and Fleck in *DRTP.*

Genetics: I pulled this information from a thesis by Ethlyn Gail Trapp, a doctoral student at the University of New South Wales. The paper, titled "Effect of High Intensity Exercise on Fat Loss in Young Overweight Women," was posted online in 2006. A study based on the research she did for her thesis will probably be published in a journal in the near future, if it hasn't already.

Genetics and exercise intensity: Bouchard et al., "Genetic effect in resting and exercise metabolic rates." *Metabolism* 1989; 38(4):364–370.

Heart-disease statistics: I got these from the American Heart Association website, mostly from a PDF file, "Heart Disease and Stroke Statistics: 2007 Update At-a-Glance."

Walking: Manson et al., "A prospective study of walking as compared with vigorous exercise in the prevention of coronary heart disease in women." *New England Journal of Medicine* 1999; 341(9):650–658. Manson et al., "Walking compared with vigorous exercise for the prevention of cardiovascular events in women." *New England Journal of Medicine* 2002; 347(10):716–725.

Chapter 4

Calorie Restriction Society: The website is calorierestriction.org. Calories typically consumed by this group were assessed in this study: Meyer et al., "Long-term caloric restriction ameliorates the decline in diastolic function in humans." *Journal of the American College of Cardiology,* 2006; 47(2):398–402.

***Calories in* Sonoma Diet:** This is from "Wine Country Diet, Sans Grape," by Sally Squires in *The Washington Post,* January 31, 2006.

Calorie restriction study: Weiss et al., "Lower extremity muscle size and strength and aerobic capacity decrease with caloric restriction but not with exercise-induced weight loss." *Journal of Applied Physiology,* e-pub ahead of print, November 9, 2006.

Cooper Institute study: Farrell et al., "The relation of body mass index, cardiorespiratory fitness, and all-cause mortality in women." *Obesity Research* 2002; 10(6):417–423.

TEF and exercise: Denzer and Young, "The effect of resistance exercise on the thermic effect of food." *International Journal of Sport Nutrition and Exercise Metabolism* 2003; 13(3):396–402. Jones et al., "Role of sympathetic neural activation in age- and habitual exercise-related differences in the thermic effect of food." *Journal of Clinical Endocrinology and Metabolism* 2004; 89(10):5138–5144.

Thinness and miscarriage: Maconochie et al., "Risk factors for first trimester miscarriage: results from a UK-population-based case-control study." *BJOG* 2007; 114(2):170–186.

Hormonal consequences of low-calorie diets: I got most of this material from the faculty page of Ohio University professor Anne Loucks, Ph.D., who's done research on the calorie needs of female athletes since the early 1990s. Dr. Loucks has sounded the alarm on the dangers of too little food for those athletes, and by extension for all women who're working out and exposing their bodies to excess stress. One of her most important points is that virtually all Americans are advised to eat less food. Our government harps on it, our diet books and magazines offer strategies to accomplish it, and our stick-figure female celebrities advertise the benefits of it every time they're filmed or photographed. The problem is that many of the women receiving this message don't actually need to eat less. As I write in Chapter 4, some should be eating more, or at least eating more at advantageous times. If my coauthors and I accomplish nothing else in this book, I hope we convince our readers that the goal of a healthy diet is to eat enough, particularly enough of the right foods at the right times. "Enough" will probably be less total food for some, but for others it could actually be more.

Chapter 5

New Food Guide Pyramid: Go to mypyramid.gov to build your own meal plan.

Diet cage match: Dansinger et al., "Comparison of the Atkins, Ornish, Weight Watchers, and Zone diets for weight loss and heart disease risk reduction: a randomized trial." *Journal of the American Medical Association* 2005; 293(1):43–53.

Higher protein versus lower protein: Astrup, "Carbohydrates as macronutrients in relation to protein and fat for body weight control." *International Journal of Obesity* 2006; 30: S4–S9. This is a review, discussing the results of several dozen studies, and advocating higher protein in combination with lower fat. Layman et al., "Dietary protein and exercise have additive effects on body composition during weight loss in adult women." *Journal of Nutrition* 2005; 135:1903–1910. This one uses higher protein in combination with lower carbohydrates. Fat was kept constant at about 30 percent of total calories.

The Good Mood Diet: This book, by Susan Kleiner, Ph.D., and Bob Condor, was released by Springboard Press in January 2007. Read more at goodmooddiet.com.

Chapter 6

Meal frequency: Farschchi et al., "Decreased thermic effect of food after an irregular compared with a regular meal pattern in healthy lean women." *International Journal of Obesity* 2004; 28(5):653–660. Louis-Sylvestre et al., "Highlighting the positive impact of increasing feeding frequency on metabolism and weight management." *Forum of Nutrition* 2003; 56:126–128. Crovetti et al., "The influence of thermic effect of food on satiety." *European Journal of Clinical Nutrition* 1998; 52(7):482–488.

Low-fat candy: Back in 1998, Ann Hodgman wrote a "Burb's Eye View" column for the June 22 issue of *Brandweek* on the emerging trend of pretending that candy offers benefits beyond the obvious. My favorite lines: "I refuse to listen to anyone who tries to persuade me that a vice is a virtue. . . . I walk away from any brand that pretends it's healthy. When I want healthy, I'll eat healthy, thank you very much. When I want candy, I want candy."

Fats and longevity: Oh et al., "Dietary fat intake and risk of coronary heart disease in women: 20 years of follow-up of the Nurses' Health Study." *American Journal of Epidemiology* 2005; 161(7):672–679.

Nuts and heart disease: Halton et al., "Low-carbohydrate-diet score and the risk of coronary heart disease in women." *New England Journal of Medicine* 2006; 355:1991–2002.

Linoleic acid and cancer: Hammamieh et al., "Differential effects of omega-3 and omega-6 fatty acids on gene expression in breast cancer cells." *Breast Cancer Research and Treatment* 2006; e-pub ahead of print. Ritch et al., "Dietary fatty acids correlate with prostate cancer biopsy grade and volume in Jamaican men." *Journal of Urology* 2007; 177(1):97–101.

Linoleic acid and obesity: Ailhaud et al., "Temporal changes in dietary fats: role of omega-6 polyunsaturated fatty acids in excessive adipose tissue development and relationship to obesity." *Progress in Lipid Research* 2006; 45:203–236.

Types of fat in animals past and present: Cordain et al., "Origins and evolution of the Western diet: Health implications for the 21st century." *American Journal of Clinical Nutrition* 2005; 81:341–354.

Balancing polyunsaturated fats: Simopoulos, "Evolutionary aspects of diet, the omega-6/omega-3 ratio and genetic variation: nutritional implications for chronic diseases." *Biomedicine & Pharmacotherapy* 2006; 60 (9):502–507.

Conjugated linoleic acid: Kim et al., "Trans-10,cis-12 conjugated linoleic acid inhibits the G1-S cell cycle progression in DU145 human prostate carcinoma cells." *Journal of Medicinal Food* 2006; 9(3):293–299. Bhattacharya et al., "Conjugated linoleic acid and chromium lower body weight and visceral fat mass in high-fat-diet-fed mice." *Lipids* 2006; 41(5):437–444. Terpstra et al., "The decrease in body fat in mice fed conjugated linoleic acid is due to increases in energy expenditure and energy loss in the excreta." *Journal of Nutrition* 2002; 132(5):940–945.

Healthy living: Key et al., "Health effects of vegetarian and vegan diets." *Proceedings of the Nutrition Society* 2006; 65(1):35–41.

Carb confusion: If you go to the *Body for Life* page on Amazon.com, you can still find the short review I wrote back in 1999. The *Washington Post* column by Sally Squires, "Mixing with a Higher Class of Carbs," was published December 19, 2006.

Fruits, vegetables, starches, etc.: As I did with *New Rules of Lifting,* I cribbed much of this material from *SuperFoods Rx* by Stephen Pratt, M.D. It remains one of my favorite books about nutrition.

Health benefits of whole grains: Slavin, "Whole grains and human health." *Nutrition Research Reviews* 2004; 17:88–110.

Argument for low protein: This was presented in "12 Simple Rules for Living Stronger," by David Walters, in the April 2006 issue of *Esquire,* on page 74. None of the tips is attributed to any single source, and at the end of the article three sources are listed: me, Chris Carmichael (Lance Armstrong's trainer and a popular author), and Marion Nestle, Ph.D., professor of nutrition, food studies, and public health at New York University and author of several books, including *Food Politics.* I'm going to guess that tip #6 ("Don't drink protein shakes. The typical American already gets more protein than even elite athletes need") came from Dr. Nestle, who published the paper "Meat or wheat for the next millennium?" *Proceedings of the Nutrition Society* 1999; 58:211–218.

Protein quality: I got this from a variety of sources, including a book called *Sports Supplements* by Jose Antonio, Ph.D., and Jeff Stout, Ph.D.

Additive effects: Wolfe, "Skeletal muscle protein metabolism and resistance exercise." *Journal of Nutrition* 2006; 136:525S–528S.

Alcohol: Westerterp, "Diet induced thermogenesis." *Nutrition & Metabolism* 2004; 1:5. Westerterp, "Alcohol energy intake and habitual physical activity in older adults." *British Journal of Nutrition* 2004; 91:149–152.

Chapter 7

Owen equation: Siervo et al., "Which REE prediction equation should we use in normal-weight, overweight and obese women?" *Clinical Nutrition* 2003; 22(2):193–204.

Calories and protein to build a pound of muscle: I got these figures from a lecture by Lonnie Lowery, Ph.D., an exercise and nutrition scientist and president of Nutrition, Exercise & Wellness Associates in Cuyahoga Falls, Ohio.

Minimal protein needs for lifters: Tarnopolsky et al., "Influence of protein intake and training status on nitrogen balance and lean body mass." *Journal of Applied Physiology* 1988; 64(1):187–193.

Chapter 8

Bodybuilding for fat loss: This is from Alwyn's *Real World Fat Loss Theory Manual*, which he released in early 2007 and which is available at alwyncosgrove.com.

The size of the pump doesn't determine the growth of the muscle: I quote from *DRTP*, page 194: "The temporary hypertrophy caused by weight training is also called the 'pump.' . . . Over time this could result in increased muscular hypertrophy. However, such speculation lacks sound supporting scientific evidence."

"Get lean, sexy legs": *Shape,* January 2007 cover.

"Firmer, more sculpted arms": Same issue of *Shape,* page 88. I should say here that *Shape* is a terrific magazine, and I hate to single it out for nitpicking. Here's why I used two examples from the same issue of the same magazine: Because it *is* a good magazine, it should be held to a higher standard; plus, imagine what the crappy ones are saying. And because it just happened to be the one I grabbed on a newsstand while I was writing this chapter. (And no, I didn't grab it just so I could nitpick it here. I buy a lot of fitness magazines.)

Chapter 9

Stuart McGill: Dr. McGill is the author of two books I've referred to often—*Low Back Disorders* (which was written for practitioners) and *Ultimate Back Fitness and Performance* (which is for a more general audience). You can check out his work at backfitpro.com.

Anatomy trains: This is from the book *Anatomy Trains,* by Thomas W. Myers. You can read more about it at anatomytrains.com. The book was published in 2001, and its subtitle tells you the intended audience: "Myofascial meridians for manual and movement therapists." In other words, we aren't talking about *Body for Life* or *YOU: The Owner's Manual.* (Although it would be entertaining to see *Myofascial Meridians for Life* or *YOU: Manipulating Your Meridians.*) I think its ideas will soon enter the conversation about exercise and fitness, just as Stuart McGill's ideas about lower-back health and safety are fast becoming conventional wisdom among trainers and other fitness professionals. McGill's original audience was people in exercise science and health care, and thanks to the fact a few geeks like me heard his lectures at sports-science conferences, his ideas soon filtered out.

I don't mean to imply that people will be talking about myofascial meridians anytime soon. The word "meridians" has been used in traditional Chinese medicine, and is unlikely to be used outside New Age circles in my lifetime. Myers's concept of meridians is anything but New Age. It's grounded in anatomy, following the directions of human connective tissues, and has real-world uses in physical therapy and injury rehabilitation.

But the word is tainted beyond hope, which is why I suspect that the idea of anatomy trains will catch on while the words in Myers's subtitle won't.

Quadriceps strength and muscle imbalance: Knapik et al., "Preseason strength and flexibility imbalances associated with athletic injuries in female collegiate athletes." *American Journal of Sports Medicine* 1991; 19(1):76–81. Ahmad et al., "Effect of gender and maturity on quadriceps-to-hamstring strength ratio and anterior cruciate ligament laxity." *American Journal of Sports Medicine* 2006; 34(3):370–374.

Chapter 11

Soviet-bloc exercises: This information comes from a short article called "From Russia . . . or Not?" which appeared on page 53 of the Fall 2004 issue of a short-lived magazine called *Muscle.* It was published by Rodale, my former employer, as a spin-off of *Men's Health* magazine. I was the magazine's original editor, but, alas, the "former" part of my Rodale tenure came during production of the magazine's second issue. Those who remember the magazine (me and maybe two or three readers) do so fondly.

Lats dance: The information about the latissimus dorsi comes from *Anatomy Trains* and *Ultimate Back Fitness and Performance.*

Hanna side flexion: These three exercises were developed by the late Thomas Hanna, Ph.D., a philosopher who became a mind-body exercise advocate and innovator. He was strongly influenced by Moshe Feldenkrais, a scientist and martial-arts aficionado who figured out a new system of movement that helped him rehabilitate a severe knee injury.

If all that sounds like gibberish, well, I'll concede the point.

But the Feldenkrais system is pretty incredible stuff. I was given a demonstration once, in the mid-1990s, by Anat Baniel, who, like Thomas Hanna, learned the system from Feldenkrais himself. After just an hour of exercises, I felt like a completely different person. One of my legs is naturally shorter than the other, but after one Feldenkrais session, they were the same length. Whatever fixed my legs also loosened my hips and pelvis to the point that I could actually dance, for the first time in my life.

I won't promise anything like those benefits from doing the side-flexion exercises, but they are interesting and different. Alwyn learned them from Paul Chek, a physical therapist and training guru based in Vista, California.

Chapter 12

Yoga, Pilates, and back pain: Williams et al., "Effect of Iyengar yoga therapy for chronic low back pain." *Pain* 2005; 115(1–2):107–117. Rydeard et al., "Pilates-based therapeutic exercise: effect on subjects with nonspecific chronic low back pain and functional disability: a randomized controlled trial." *Journal of Orthopaedic & Sports Physical Therapy,* 2006; 36(7):472–484.

Chapter 13

Choices: This entire discussion was inspired by a conversation with my friend Charles Staley, a strength coach based in Phoenix. I'd guess it was sometime in 2003, give or take a year. Charles said that he used to tell people he had a goal of hitting a particular personal record in a particular exercise. But after a few years, he realized that he hadn't done anything concrete to reach that goal. Therefore, it wasn't really a goal, since he wasn't working his way toward it in any meaningful way. He downgraded the goal of a personal record to "fantasy" or "daydream" status, and he was totally fine with that. After all, not choosing to accomplish something is still a choice.

Now is as good a time as any to note that *The New Rules of Lifting for Women* is chock-full of ideas and insights I've picked up from my fellow travelers in the fitness world. I've tried to acknowledge where ideas come from to the best of my memory, but my memory is imperfect. So I'd like to thank everyone whose knowledge and analytical skills inspired the material in this book, while apologizing in advance to all those who didn't receive credit where it was surely due.

Index